The

FOOD ALLERGY EXPERIENCE

Real voices. Real disease. Real insights.

RUCHI GUPTA MD, MPH

With special contribution from
Denise A. Bunning

Comic Illustrations by
Tiffany Glass Ferreira

ISBN: 1480027537
ISBN-13: 9781480027534

Library of Congress Control Number: 2012912111
CreateSpace, North Charleston, SC

ACKNOWLEDGMENTS

Special thanks to all the parents, doctors,
teachers, researchers, and advocates who contributed to this book

Sarah Boudreau-Romano, MD
Carmen-Rae Carlson
Liliana DeSantiago
Caroline Duda
Ashley Dyer, MPH
Mary Pat Dyer
Raina Gupta, MD
Reshma Jagsi-Pottow, MD
Tarun Jain, MD
Jennifer Jobrack
Donna Kaufman
Sugeeta Kohli
Michelle Knight
Claudia Lau
Sean McGill
Bela Mehta
Michael Pistiner, MD, MMSc
Sheila Raja, PhD
Lauren Scalzo
Jessica Severino
Elizabeth Springston
Christine Szychlinski, APN, NP
Anne Thompson
Karen M. Thorne
Chef Dominique Tougne

Elena Turczeniuk
Chris Warren
Manoj Warrier, MD
Lauren Lowe
Jeanette Washington
Stephanie Whyte, MD, MPH
Amy Wicker

...And many more

*To my husband Tarun, our parents, our friends, and
our children Rohan and Riya*

CONTENTS

Preface   ix
Introduction   xi

PART ONE: THE BEGINNING   1

  1. Reactions   3
  2. Diagnosis   11
  3. Treatment   17
  4. Finances   25
  5. Advocating for Your Child   31
  6. Public Policy   41

PART TWO: RELATIONSHIPS   47

  7. Support Systems   49
  8. Marriage and Relationships   53
  9. Family   59
  10. Friends   65
  11. My Doctor   71

PART THREE: SOCIAL WORLD   77

  12. Day Care and School   79
  13. Social Activities   91
  14. Dining Out   99
  15. Traveling   107
  16. Isolation   113

PART FOUR: EVERYDAY   **119**

17. Daily Life   121
18. Meals and Nutrition   127
19. Feeling Different   135
20. The Parent's Emotions   141
21. The Child's Emotions   151
22. Transitions and Growing Up   157
23. Success Stories   165

Final Thoughts   169
Resources   171
References   183

PREFACE

food allergy (fud ˈæl.ɚ.dʒi) *n.* "An adverse health effect arising from a specific immune response that occurs reproducibly on exposure to a given food."

Guidelines for the Diagnosis and Management of Food Allergy in the United States: Summary of the NIAID sponsored Expert Panel Report, Boyce et al., 2010

- Food allergy affects 5.9 million, or 8 percent, of children in the United States.[1] This is one in thirteen children, or two children per classroom.

- Individuals can be diagnosed with a food allergy from birth to adulthood.

- Almost 4 percent of children with food allergy have experienced a severe, life-threatening reaction from an accidental food ingestion.[1]

- Children of all ages are most allergic to peanuts, milk, shellfish, tree nuts, eggs, fin fish, wheat, soy, and sesame.[1]

- Researchers are working hard to find a cure for food allergy.

- Strict avoidance, proper symptom identification, and swift treatment are the current mainstays of food allergy management.

- Treatment involves a quick response with an epinephrine auto-injector to treat a severe reaction that can potentially lead to death. For less severe reactions, antihistamines are used.

- The majority of food allergy reactions occur away from home. About 76 percent of food allergy-related *deaths* are due to foods eaten outside the home.

- Food allergy can be confusing and overwhelming for the child, parents, friends, family, and caregivers.[2-6]

- Fortunately, we are learning more every day and gaining a better understanding of food allergy, including the causes and the treatments.

INTRODUCTION

"One of the most valuable things we can do to heal one another is listen to each other's stories." - Rebecca Falls

This book is a compilation of many people's stories. Here is mine. When I decided to specialize in pediatrics after medical school, I did it for the love of children and the potential ability to improve their lives and those of their families. Following my pediatric training, I completed a special fellowship in Boston to gain research skills in order to make a broader impact. Completion of this training opened the door for me to work with a world expert in pediatric asthma. During this time, I met a family who was passionate about the state of another related pediatric condition, "food allergy." This family would influence my work and my career dramatically. Their interest, with its deep commitment and personal stories, became my passion.

As I started working as a pediatrician and food allergy researcher, I spent time with many parents of children with food allergy. I was deeply moved by the impact of food allergy on the children and their families. Since food is a part of almost everything we do, families were affected all the time and everywhere. Keeping kids safe from allergenic food was the mission. Safe from food—that sounds so strange. This is why food allergy became such an all-encompassing issue. Care was needed everywhere a child was—at home, school, camp, friends' homes, families' homes, vacations, restaurants... everywhere.

Little did I know that I would also join the group of families having a child with food allergy. After working in this field for a few years, my daughter was born, and she was soon diagnosed with egg, peanut, and tree nut allergies. My older son, however, was allergy-free. I now experience firsthand everything parents told me. My kids live different lives. My son is worry-free when eating. We work hard to keep my daughter safe at school, during sports, at camp, and when she is with her friends or extended family. I started with the perspective of a physician and researcher, and have now added the personal experience and feelings of a parent whose child has food allergies.

The idea to write this book came during a talk I gave at a food allergy support group meeting. Prior to the meeting, I had conducted an extensive survey on the knowledge, attitudes, and beliefs surrounding food allergy among parents of children with food allergy. The parents took the time to fill up the comments section of the survey with detailed stories of their food allergy experience. I subsequently started compiling these and other stories from parents and children. I presented some of these stories at the support group meeting, and the response was overwhelming. All the parents empathized with the stories and asked if I could provide the quotes to them in a book to help them and others understand all aspects of life with a food-allergic child. In the last two years, we gathered additional quotes, tips and resources from parents, doctors, and teachers to compile this book on the food allergy experience. We added the comics to lighten the mood, because although food allergy is a very serious issue, we all need to be able to smile and laugh.

I hope this book helps families living with food allergy and helps all the people involved in a child's life better understand what that child's day-to-day world is like and what it takes to keep them safe. My daughter, who happens to have food allergies, is amazing, and our life is beautiful with her. This book is for all the children around the world with food allergy and for the people involved in their lives.

With the support of families and the hard work of researchers, I believe we will have a cure in the near future. Until then, the goal is to have understanding, love, and support among everyone who cares for our children.

Ruchi S. Gupta, MD, MPH

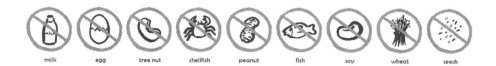

milk egg tree nut shellfish peanut fish soy wheat seeds

I was very excited to be asked to participate in a book about the experience of living with food allergy. Not only is the subject near and dear to my heart, but it's also a reality that my family has lived with for eighteen years. I believe that having the support of other food-allergic families is crucial to navigating and thriving with food allergies. So a book that features stories from many food-allergic families can only serve to encourage and motivate others who live with this daily challenge; and I'm thrilled to share my experience as well.

I've always loved children. In college I majored in early childhood/special education. I got a master's in special education and then another master's in school administration (yes, I love school). I taught second and third grade, and my plan was to become a principal. But life had a different plan for me.

After struggling for years to have my first child, I was lucky enough to be a stay-at-home mom. I nursed exclusively for six months, at which time the doctors said that if I wanted to try for another child, I'd better get going. I decided that meant I needed to start weaning my son. So, one morning after my husband left for work and I was still dressed in my pajamas, I excitedly phoned my mom so we could "feed the baby together." I gave my son his first sip of a bottle of a milk-based formula. To my horror, I watched his lips and tongue swell and his eyes roll back in his head. He turned bright red.

I screamed, "Mom, something's wrong with the baby!"

She said, "Hang up and call 911!"

But we lived in a high-rise apartment in the city, and I knew finding the building was confusing, so I grabbed my cell phone and the baby's car seat and rushed down the elevator, praying a cab would be waiting. It was, and I gratefully hopped in, and we raced to the pediatrician's office.

When I got there, I flagged a nurse, yelling frantically, "Please help my baby!"

The nurse looked at him and said, "What did you give him?"

"One sip of formula," was my only answer.

They whisked him away and said, "He's having a severe allergic reaction. We are going to give him some Benadryl, and he may need a shot of epinephrine." Minutes seemed like hours. When he finally "deflated," the nurse said, "We've never seen such a serious reaction. You need to go see a pediatric allergist right away."

This experience and the following diagnosis changed my life.

After first being introduced to *anaphylaxis* so dramatically that day eighteen years ago, we've been through many nerve-wrecking experiences: my older son's diagnosis of life-threatening food allergies to milk, eggs, tree nuts, and sesame; a variety of reactions from mild to severe; several food challenges; a diagnosis of environmental allergies and asthma at age seven; "winning the lottery" as he outgrew his milk allergy contrasted with needing two doses of EPI during a subsequent egg challenge, both at age eleven; and most recently outgrowing his egg allergy at age seventeen.

My younger son's story has been even more challenging: an initial diagnosis of his life-threatening food allergies to milk, egg, tree nuts, shellfish, and beef as an infant; a variety of reactions from mild to severe; outgrowing his egg allergy at age six; being diagnosed with environmental allergies at age seven and, more seriously, with eosinophilic esophagitis (EoE) at age nine; the insertion of a gastric tube at age ten so he could be tube fed; and more than fifteen endoscopies. And the process continues.

In 1997, feeling isolated and baffled as a parent of two kids with life-threatening food allergies (especially to milk and eggs), I wanted to start a support group. Fortunately, another mom in a nearby town was also interested. So together we founded MOCHA: Mothers of Children Having Allergies. What began as several moms getting together to discuss life with food allergies has become an organization of more than 350 families and has spawned numerous additional community-based support groups. Our goal was to provide a forum for families living with this diagnosis. I believe it is vitally important for families to connect with others who "get it" and to develop a network of resources as they navigate the many challenges that accompany this disease.

I believe this book can be an important resource to encourage food-allergic families and to educate others we know who need to learn about the surprisingly extensive effects of living with food allergy.

I am excited and hopeful about the recent news of the two national food allergy organizations merging. It means that more researchers, allergists, pediatricians, nurses, support group leaders, elected officials, administrators, teachers, parents, community members, and children can share their knowledge with each other more effectively. It validates what I strongly believe: that if we all work together (and I mean *all* of us), we can create a better life for food-allergic children and their families.

I look forward to the day in the not-so-distant future when food allergies are no longer life threatening and the complications of the disease itself are a distant memory. Until then, we will work towards a *cure*.

As for now, educate yourself, stay positive, and as I always say, "Stay Safe!"

Denise A. Bunning
MOCHA Co-Founder

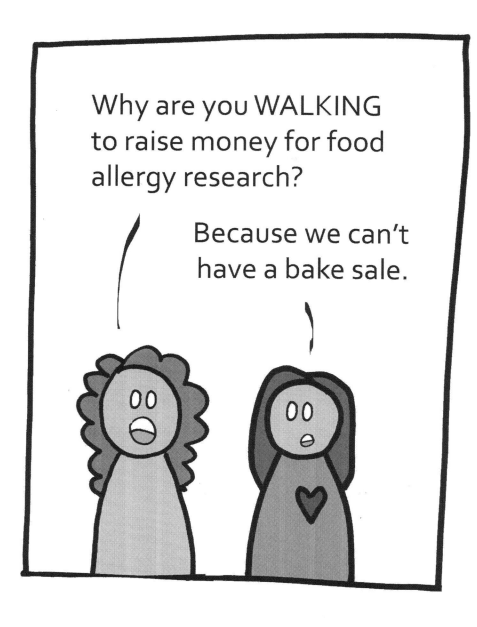

PART ONE:
THE BEGINNING

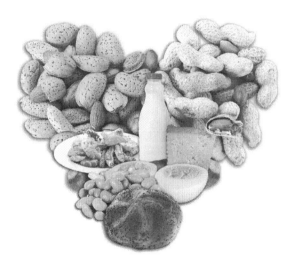

Childhood food allergy is a *serious* and *growing* health problem in the United States and much of the world

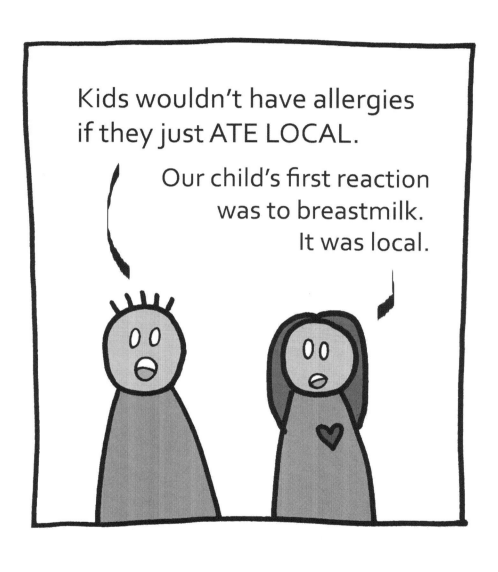

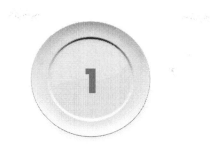

REACTIONS

anaphylaxis (ˌænəfəˈlæksɪs) *n.* A serious allergic reaction that is rapid in onset and may cause death.

Guidelines for the Diagnosis and Management of Food Allergy in the United States: Summary of the NIAID-sponsored Expert Panel Report, Boyce et al., 2010

Mild symptoms may include:

MOUTH:	Itchy mouth
SKIN:	A few hives around mouth/face/body, swelling of lips, eyes, face, mild itch
GUT:	Mild nausea/discomfort

Severe symptoms may include **one or more** of the following:

LUNG:	Shortness of breath, wheeze, repetitive cough
HEART:	Pale, blue, faint, weak pulse, dizzy, confused
THROAT:	Tight, hoarse, trouble breathing/swallowing
MOUTH:	Obstructive swelling (e.g., tongue and/or lips)
SKIN:	Many hives over body

Or, **combination** of symptoms from different body areas:

SKIN: Hives, itchy rashes, swelling (e.g., eyes, lips)
GUT: Vomiting, diarrhea, crampy pain

Food allergy is different from food intolerance. Food allergy is an immune system response while food intolerance is a digestive system response. An example of food intolerance is lactose intolerance. A person is unable to breakdown the lactose in milk and develops GI irritation. This is different from a milk allergy which is immune mediated and can result in the symptoms above.

Food allergy reactions can range from mild to life-threatening. Unfortunately, there is no way to tell what type of reaction a child will have when exposed to an allergenic food. Even if a child has had mild reactions in the past, he or she can have a severe reaction any time. More troubling, *any* allergenic food can cause a severe, life-threatening reaction. A mild reaction may require an antihistamine like Benadryl, Claritin, Zyrtec, or Allegra. A severe reaction will require an epinephrine injection (EpiPen or Twinject), sometimes as soon as minutes after exposure to a food.

Two out of five food-allergic children (40 percent) have had a severe reaction.[1] Severe reactions are most common among children with multiple food allergies or children with a confirmed sesame, shellfish, tree nut, or peanut allergy.[1] Severe reactions are also most common among teenagers.[1] This is likely due to an increase in risk-taking behavior and less parental monitoring. With proper diagnosis and understanding of the risks, food allergy is manageable throughout daily life.

• • •

"A few weeks ago my child had a peanut reaction at home to a food that should have been safe, and now she seems to be getting a hive or two quite often, which is a source of worry every time it happens. This is a more stressful time than usual."

• • •

"Looking back on his first reaction to a chocolate walnut bar was heart breaking and comical. 'Delicious' was followed by a puzzled look and 'I can't get the taste out.' I quickly glanced at my wife, who then said, 'You're such an allergist. He's just got a piece caught at the back of his mouth.' Vomiting soon occurred in the fish department of our local grocery store, where a very annoyed employee encouraged us to take him to the dingy bathroom in the back. For me, any reservations in calling this an allergic reaction were gone after we stunk up the fish department even more, but my wife, even after some irritability and throat clearing, didn't buy it until he had hives. Then she looked at me and said, 'I think he's having an allergic reaction.'"

• • •

"Although my son has many food allergies, I worry most about the dairy, as he is well trained to not touch, accept, or eat any food without first asking me. But I cannot always control who 'touches' him. Thankfully, thus far, all reactions by contact have mostly resulted in superficial symptoms, including hives and facial swelling."

• • •

"One of my sons has had two anaphylactic reactions, and it never leaves you. You cannot ever forget. It's like a broken record...just the feverishness, and this helplessness—horrible helplessness—a feeling you cannot describe. It is such a gut-wrenching squeezing of your body when you see your child going through that."

• • •

5

"We were at my in-laws, and my son accidentally grabbed a real ice cream bar instead of the soy version. He ate a few bites, came over to me, and said he did not feel well. His ears were bright red, and his lip was starting to swell. We realized what happened and gave him Benadryl. Then he said his chest hurt, and he started vomiting. At this point, his face was red, and he was covered in hives. The Benadryl was not working, and in all honesty, I should have done the EpiPen right away. Brock was crying and begging me not to. Anyway, I did give him the EpiPen and called 911. The ambulance got here very quickly, gave him an IV, and started monitoring his vitals. They took us to the nearest hospital, which luckily has a pediatric ER. They gave him more Benadryl, steroids, fluids, and a breathing treatment. He is okay now. We are all understandably freaked out but super grateful for the EpiPen and the great medical care he received."

• • •

"My child can get an allergic reaction if he comes into contact with others who eat the allergenic foods. This includes hugs, shaking hands, doorknobs, handles...everything. We keep him safe at home, but this greatly limits us in public places, all of which revolve around food and consumption."

• • •

"My daughter was six when I had to use the EpiPen on her the very first time. She was exhibiting multiple symptoms – throat swelling, bad stomach ache and large hives. I knew I had no choice. She was scared, and we both cried as I stuck the EpiPen into her leg. When I pulled it out, she said to me, 'Is that it?' Within seconds, she then said, 'Wow, I feel so much better.'"

TIPS

"Do what you can, with what you have, where you are."
- Theodore Roosevelt

✓ **Accidents happen.** Reduce the risk of a reaction and know how to treat one.

✓ **Review the details of an allergic reaction with your allergist soon after the event.** You may forget important details about the trigger or treatment approach as time passes. Make sure that you understand it.

✓ **Watch food-allergic children for not only physical but also *behavioral* and *emotional* signs of a reaction.** Behavioral signs include sudden fatigue or social withdrawal. Emotional signs include sudden crying or increased anxiety. (This is especially important to explain to your child's teachers or caregivers, as this is often the first symptom.)

✓ **Be aware of the details of allergic reactions that the child has had in the past,** and share these with people who will be taking care of your child when you are not there.

✓ Know the symptoms of an allergic reaction (www.faiusa.org).

✓ Teach your children to keep their hands out of their mouth, eyes, and nose.

✓ Have your child wear a medical identification bracelet or necklace where paramedics can see it.

What happens when someone eats an allergenic food:

The food that one is allergic to enters the body. It finds its way to allergic cells (mast cells and basophils) that recognize only certain foods through their immunoglobulin E (IgE) antibodies. Once the allergenic food protein binds to that IgE, the cell pours out chemicals (histamine and tryptase) that cause swelling, itching, decreased blood pressure, and possibly death. Epinephrine counteracts these effects. It decreases swelling, increases blood pressure, makes the heart pump better, and helps to prevent a fatal reaction.

What to do if someone is experiencing anaphylaxis:

Injectable epinephrine must be given immediately. **Be a hero. Save a life. Don't be afraid.** Once you give the injectable epinephrine as instructed, here is what it does:

Epinephrine (also known as adrenaline) constricts blood vessels. This is important because it curbs the microvascular leaking that leads to decreased blood volume and plummeting blood pressure, which can lead to shock and death. Epinephrine relaxes airways. So, while histamine is causing airways to swell and tighten up, epinephrine helps to decrease swelling in the upper airway so that air is not obstructed from getting to the lungs. Epinephrine also decreases cramping of the gastrointestinal tract and helps to block the hives and itching that accompany an allergic reaction.

Epinephrine can help to stop anaphylaxis from progressing to death if given early and appropriately. It is the *only* thing that can. Antihistamines, like Benadryl or Claritin, can relieve some of the skin symptoms (hives, itching) but they *do not* have the ability to save a life from anaphylaxis.

For an excellent, in-depth explanation, visit www.theallergistmom. com.

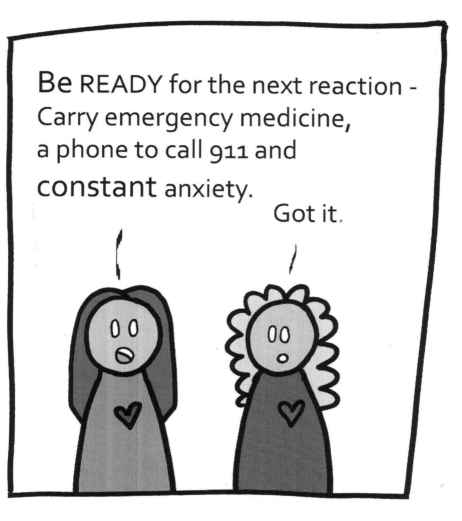

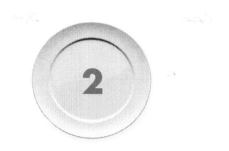

DIAGNOSIS

oral food challenge (ˈɔːɹəl fud ˈtʃæl.ɪndʒ) *n.* A test where the patient eats specific foods under medical supervision to determine if the individual has an allergy to that food.

Diagnosis of a food allergy usually starts when a child reacts negatively to a food. A health-care provider (pediatrician, family physician, allergist, or nurse practitioner) will take a history of the reaction and conduct some initial testing, which could include a skin prick test or a blood test for the IgE (the antibody elicited by an allergic substance like the allergenic food). Interpreting these tests must be done with a health-care provider, as the results of the testing with clinical history determine suggested management.

The most reliable test for diagnosing a food allergy or determining if a child has outgrown an allergy (developed tolerance) is called an *oral food challenge.* During an oral food challenge, the doctor carefully observes the child while he or she consumes increasing amounts of an allergenic food. If the child has had a reaction to a food and the tests are positive, we consider the child to be allergic. A child should have testing done with the specific foods they reacted to and not to foods they currently eat and tolerate well.

Guidelines for the diagnosis and management of food allergies were recently published and can be accessed at the National Institute of Allergy and Infectious Diseases website:

http://www.niaid.nih.gov/topics/foodAllergy/clinical/Pages/patients.aspx

• • •

"My child suffered from food allergies practically from birth. She developed severe eczema by three months and was diagnosed with food allergies in her first year."

• • •

"I have worries that he may develop new, more serious allergies, despite scores of zero on both the RAST (blood IgE) and skin prick tests."

• • •

"My son is nearly seven; he was diagnosed with his food allergies right after his first birthday (dairy and eggs)."

• • •

"I just got poor results from my child's yearly testing (skin prick test and RAST), and then my child had an unexplained reaction (for the fourth time) at preschool due to an unidentified cause."

• • •

"I have had a hard week because my son just got his blood test results back this week. He is almost seven and has not outgrown any of his allergies, according to the blood test."

• • •

"My elder son was just diagnosed with allergies to tree nuts and soy at the age of 17. I'm very fearful of him leaving for college."

• • •

"We were so happy when he outgrew his milk allergy, but then when he ate peanut he got so sick, he needed epinephrine. We were so sure we could put food allergy behind us, but are we being ungrateful? At least he can drink milk now."

TIPS

"We must constantly build dykes of courage to hold back the flood of fear."
- Martin Luther King Jr.

How can a parent prepare for the news of a child's diagnosis?

✓ **The best thing a parent can do is to stay on the safe side.** If you think something might be wrong with your child, find a health-care provider you trust to conduct an evaluation. Educate yourself.

✓ **Reflect on how you've coped with difficult times before, and try to use some of those positive coping skills now.** Whether it is yoga, prayer, talking to friends, or reading magazines to distract yourself— do something to help you cope with your short-term anxiety.

✓ **Every time you go to a health-care provider, prepare yourself and your child for whatever the results may show.** Remind yourself that you and your child can learn to deal with the results, one day at a time.

✓ **Join a food allergy support group and talk to other parents.**

✓ **Don't trust everything on the Internet.** Make sure you are reading from a reputable website. Ask your doctor or allergist which websites are the most useful.

✓ **Become an advocate for your child.** Try not to focus on the negative; instead focus your energies on learning about food allergies and the best way to help your child lead a fulfilling life. Keeping busy learning and adapting will help you avoid negative thoughts and despair.

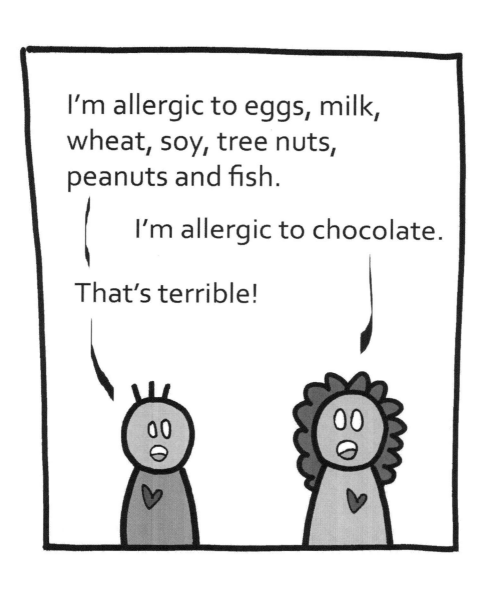

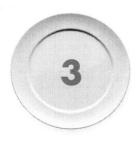

TREATMENT

epinephrine (ɛprˈnɛfɪn) *n.* A hormone that can prevent fatal anaphylaxis upon prompt administration, but only when adverse reactions are recognized in a timely manner.

There is no proven cure for food allergy, nor are there any medications that prevent food allergy reactions. Allergen avoidance is the first and only line of prevention.

A common misconception among the public is that there is already a cure for food allergy.[4] Parents of food-allergic children may have to educate friends and family about these misconceptions.

It is critical that caregivers be able to recognize early signs of food allergy reactions. If the reaction is mild, like a rash (hives), a caregiver may give an antihistamine (Benadryl, Claritin, Zyrtec, or Allegra).

If the child looks like he or she is having a severe reaction (trouble breathing, throat getting tight, wheezing, drop in blood pressure, feeling faint, etc.) the caregiver should inject epinephrine (EpiPen, Twinject) in the outside thigh and hold it there for 10 seconds. The caregiver or a helper should also call 911 and the child's parents immediately. If the child does not look like he or she is improving, a second dose of epinephrine may be needed. Talk to your child's doctor about exactly what you should do in case of a food-induced emergency.

New studies are being conducted on immunotherapy, which is the gradual introduction of an allergenic food to the allergic individual's diet over time as a possible treatment or cure. This is still in the research phase, but does hold promise. Other treatments are also being tested using alternative therapies. Researchers are working hard to find a cure.

• • •

"I definitely would like more education on having, carrying, and using an EpiPen and anaphylaxis. Just because the doctor pre-scribes it and you carry it, does not mean you feel equipped to know when it needs to be used and when not to use it."

• • •

"It is so important that we (parents) choose our words wisely around our children. I have witnessed so many parents saying how badly an auto-injector hurts or how long the needle is, without themselves experiencing it. Remember that kids believe what we tell them. We should be honest but think about ways to do this with-out terrifying. My son's perception is that 'the needle is short and skinny, and the medicine makes you feel better really fast.'"

• • •

"I have four kids, so I am trying to answer for all of them. But my seven-year-old has so many food allergies and EoE [eosinophilic esophagitis], that he has a g-tube now and only gets Neocate Jr... so he is on the extreme end of how food allergies run our lives."

• • •

"I am a physician and can handle a medical emergency but could not give my own child epinephrine when it was needed."

• • •

"As a parent who has had to use an EpiPen on her fourteen-month-old for a severe allergic reaction to eggs, I want other parents to know that they should trust their instincts and not be afraid to use the epinephrine just because they think it might hurt the child. The pain of an injection is likely much less than the severe discomfort your child may be experiencing due to trouble breathing and other symptoms. If you think that your child may need epinephrine, use it."

• • •

"Now that my son is four, we are asking him to practice with a *practice* EpiPen on himself. Ultimately, his knowledge is the best prevention against a reaction. We also have asked our nanny and extended family to train themselves with the EpiPen."

• • •

"We carry EpiPens at all time and have one stored at school, at grandparents' homes, and in the backpack. Just knowing they are within reach gives us comfort."

• • •

"I carry an EpiPen, but I wish people didn't think that makes it okay not to be careful to avoid nuts. So they'll say things like, 'What are you so worried about? If there's a little bit of nut in the food, you have an EpiPen, don't you?' They don't seem to realize that even with an EpiPen administered promptly, there can be serious outcomes."

• • •

"I didn't realize there was a psychological barrier because I had never used the EpiPen before. Once you get past that first time, you won't be as afraid of it, and you'll be more willing to use it."

TIPS

"True freedom lies in the realization and calm acceptance of the fact that there may very well be no perfect answer."
- Allen Reid McGinnis

✓ **Know when to administer life-saving medication.** Review the emergency protocol that your allergist gives you. Make certain that you can explain it to other caregivers, such as teachers, school nurses, and bus drivers.

✓ **Practice performing injections into an orange using an expired epinephrine auto-injector.** The more you practice using it, the more confident you will be if you have to use one during an emergency.

✓ **Make sure all caregivers know what to do if your child has an allergic reaction.** They may not be able to reach you, and you cannot assess a situation over the phone.

✓ **Consider training others using an expired epinephrine auto-injector** such as your child, your child's teacher, caregivers, and siblings.

✓ **Some children get hives. Others do not.** Discuss with your doctor what your child's allergic features are, understand them, and make sure caregivers know how to recognize the first signs of an allergic reaction in progress.

✓ **Be sure not to place your thumb over the end of the auto-injector;** you might puncture your thumb with the needle. If this happens, seek emergency care.

✓ **Emergency medication.** In every kit carry:
  - Printed emergency protocol
  - Two epinephrine auto-injectors (no trainer)
  - Liquid Benadryl (if using single servings, pre-open the wrapper)
  - Wipes
  - Safe snack
  - Money

✓ **Don't leave home without it; a reaction can occur when you least expect it.** Keep medicine kits and copies of your emergency protocol everywhere you may need them. You do not want to have to leave your child alone while you go in search of an epinephrine auto-injector.

✓ **Most schools are equipped with a procedure to address a food-induced emergency.** Ask your school if your child's teacher and school staff are properly trained to help. If not, take it upon yourself to set up a training session with a local hospital or nurse practitioner.

✓ **Training resources are available through organizations like the Food Allergy Initiative (www.faiusa.org) and the Food Allergy & Anaphylaxis Network (www.foodallergy.org).** Training modules to assist in training other caregivers in various settings (relatives, babysitters, schools, camps, etc.) can be found at AllergyHome.org. You can also ask local support groups for assistance.

✓ **If you encounter someone who has had to give an epinephrine injection, let him or her tell the story uninterrupted.** It will help him or her and help you.

✓ Whenever you change your clocks, check your child's epinephrine auto-injector and emergency medication's expiration dates to
ensure they are still valid.

✓ Make sure to hold the epinephrine auto-injector in the lateral
(outer) thigh for ten seconds before removing it. When you administer the auto-injector and when you remove it, you and the child will
never see the needle, as it is covered. Also remember that you can and
should inject through a layer of clothing.

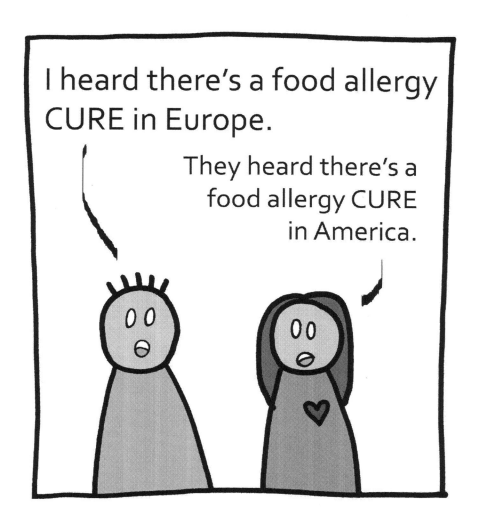

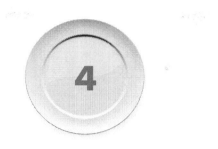

FINANCES

allergen-free (ˈælərdʒən) *n.* Without the food or substance that the child is allergic to.

Food allergy can put strains on caregivers' finances. Mothers, in particular, have stopped working or changed jobs to stay closer to home to keep their children safer by monitoring their food intake in school and at home.[2] In addition to reduced income, families of children with severe food allergy reactions are often burdened with the extra cost of office visit copayments, other out-of-pocket medical bills, medicines, and special allergen-free foods.[7] Overall, parents report spending an additional 4,700 dollars per year due to expenses related to food allergy.[7]

• • •

"Life is very challenging because I take his care as a full-time job. I haven't gone back to work since having him, and that wasn't the initial plan."

• • •

"I have had to quit my job so that I can be available for any needs, whether it is a school party, a field trip, afterschool activities, etc. I have the time now to shop, make calls, cook, prepare, research, etc., which is a lot of work."

• • •

We must have lost at least 150 dollars worth the day my wife and I looked in our cabinets and started sorting out all the food with advisory statements for tree nuts. The items that we now get tend to be significantly more expensive than if we could shop without avoiding his allergens."

• • •

"This year, the PTA decided to give parents the opportunity to have a chocolate sucker delivered to their child in their classroom on Valentine's Day. I had to hurry and order a peanut-free holiday sucker from a website and pay seven dollars in shipping for a one-dollar sucker so my daughter will not feel left out when other children get their suckers. This on top of the actual holiday classroom party is killing me as a full-time, working mother of two."

• • •

"We have created a very safe environment for our child, involving constant supervision and extensive child care. We are concerned that most other families cannot afford this support."

• • •

"This stress affects my work, my marriage, my parenting skills, and my outlook on life. Due to my son's peanut allergy, we are forced to place him in a peanut-free private school at significant cost to us."

• • •

"The allergies played a role in my decision to leave work, and they played a role in deciding what school my daughter would attend. It seems to be a factor in most of what we do as a family."

• • •

"I cannot afford visits to the allergist and dermatologist, even though my son's skin is terrible due to his allergies. I think he may have other undiagnosed allergies, but at this point, we cannot afford more visits and lab fees to find out. In addition, I really feel the need to visit a nutritionist or a dietician who specializes in children with food allergies, but resources for that are limited in this community, and we can't afford a trip to the big city and the medical bills."

• • •

"Our biggest stresses are the costs of feeding our children certain foods that don't make them sick."

• • •

"Either you reduce your work hours to take the time to make all meals from scratch yourself, or you have to start paying top dollar for the few prepared foods that are safe."

TIPS

"I've failed over and over and over again in my life,
and that is why I succeed."
- Michael Jordan

✓ **Plan ahead.** Stock safe foods for impromptu parties.

✓ **Talk to other families** to get information on local or online resources.

✓ **Make a food calendar.** If you plan ahead for every meal for one week, and repeat weekly, you will be better prepared at the grocery store. When you learn of new recipes, you can create an additional list and switch out items on your calendar.

✓ **Avoid prepared foods.** Instead of buying boxes of prepared foods, read the ingredients and buy each ingredient separately. Usually your money will go much further.

✓ **Remember that what kids like can be simple.** If you make or buy some of your kids' favorite treats, that may be enough to keep them happy. Often kids do not need endless variety to feel satisfied and included.

✓ **Check to see if you qualify** to deduct the costs of gluten- or other allergen-free foods from your income taxes. IRS Publication 502, Medical and Dental Expenses, addresses food deductions related to *weight-loss* diets (not specifically allergen-free diets). Language in this

IRS publication states that deductions (again, for medically prescribed weight-loss diets) apply when "The food alleviates or treats an illness, and disease (and) the need for the food is substantiated by a physician." The amount you can include in medical expenses is limited to the amount by which the cost of the special food exceeds the cost of a normal diet.

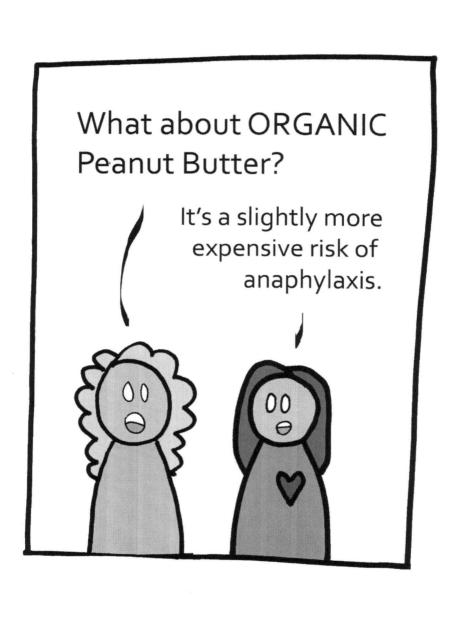

ADVOCATING FOR YOUR CHILD

FAAN (fæn) *n.* Food Allergy & Anaphylaxis Network.
FAI (ɛf,eɪ,aɪ) *n.* Food Allergy Initiative.

Seventy-six percent of food allergy-related deaths are due to foods eaten outside the home. Our community plays an important role in ensuring the well-being of children with food allergy, whether at restaurants, entertainment facilities such as movie theaters, schools, or child-care facilities. Our research has found that the general community is often unaware that there is no cure for food allergy and there is no daily medication that can prevent an allergic reaction.[4] This is important to know when advocating for your child.

Improving your community's knowledge of prevention, symptoms, and treatment can save a child's life. Organizations like the Food Allergy & Anaphylaxis Network *(FAAN)* and the Food Allergy Initiative

(*FAI*) as well as local parent support groups can offer multiple resources to help raise awareness in your community.

The Food Allergy & Anaphylaxis Network (FAAN) is the world leader in information, resources, and programs for food allergy. A national nonprofit organization based in Virginia, FAAN is dedicated to increasing public awareness of food allergy and its consequences, educating people about the condition, and advancing research on behalf of all those affected by it. FAAN provides educational resources about food allergy to patients, families, schools, health professionals, pharmaceutical companies, the food industry, and government officials.

The Food Allergy Initiative (FAI) is the world's largest source of private funding for food allergy research. A national nonprofit based in New York, FAI's goal is to fund research that seeks a cure, improve diagnosis and treatment, increase federal funding of food allergy research, create safer environments through advocacy, and raise awareness through education.

On May 9, 2012, FAAN and FAI announced their intent to merge, pending state regulatory approval. The unified organization will focus on funding research to find a cure, advocating for food-allergic people, increasing awareness about the severity and growing prevalence of food allergies, and educating the public and other key stakeholders about the disease and the urgent need for a cure. (www.foodallergy.org)

• • •

"Never in these years has my child been surrounded by adults in authority who know more or even as much as my child and our family. ... We are constantly vigilant and educating others to keep our child safe."

• • •

"It is like speaking but not having a voice. Silence. Stares. They don't want to hear, and I know someone is going to die on that campus in the coming years... They are not ready."

• • •

"One approach is to attempt community-wide education that comes from sources like school nurses, teachers, doctors, educators, and advocacy groups that may take some of the pressure and onus off parents. With time, we may find that our educated communities continue a cycle of awareness that makes it easier and easier for parents to educate others about caring for their specific child's allergies. There will be less reinventing the wheel, as well as less resistance and skepticism."

• • •

"My anxieties have lessened due to advocating in the schools for my allergic kids, which has empowered me. The schools have stepped up and trained personnel, which has made things better for everyone."

• • •

"Everybody should be informed that food allergies can kill, and we should teach our children never to share food or snacks. My son knows the seriousness of his allergy. He knows he can die if he eats eggs. We have a saying in our house when it comes to not knowing if egg is an ingredient in a particular food: when in doubt, do without."

• • •

"My daughter with nut allergy is now old enough to read labels to double-check ingredients. The school's safety procedures for her have steadily improved over the last three years due to lots of work on my part. She now has a 504 plan (a plan developed by a parent and school to protect the child with a disability or chronic illness) in place, which has seemed to help. But the process of educating staff and parents is never ending."

• • •

"I overheard a coworker talking about how she really 'hates those crazy nut allergy moms.' I'm friendly with her, so I said, 'You do realize that I have a child with a nut allergy, right?' Her response was, 'Oh, yeah, but I'm sure you're not annoying like the mom in my kid's class. Every year, at the first big parent meeting, she reminds us that her kid has a nut allergy. My own kid has learning disabilities, but I don't waste other parents' time telling them about that every year. I just don't understand why parents with kids with allergies seem to think they have the right to bother other parents about it.' I tried to be nice and explain how hard it is to know that your child can lose her life in a moment if someone unknowingly feeds her something with a trace of a nut. It's not quite the same as a learning disability, though community is clearly important in both cases. We need our neighbors to help us keep these kids safe, but we have to be so careful about how we do it so that we don't alienate them in our well-intentioned attempts to ask for their help."

• • •

"My daughter, who is anaphylactic to milk, eggs and all nuts, came home from junior kindergarten one day and told me that she had done an experiment involving M&Ms. Never before had she even touched an M&M. She said that the teacher made her take one and soak it in some water. She knew she wasn't supposed to be handling it, but she was doing what the teacher had asked her. I knew then how important it was for her to know that it was okay to say no to a teacher or authority figure if she thought it would put her in danger. No one knows her allergies better than she does."

TIPS

"Do not wait for leaders; do it alone, person to person."
- Mother Teresa

✓ **Don't be afraid to approach and educate the people who you are trusting with your child's life.** Do your own due diligence—*every time*. Keep in mind that your child's tolerance level may be different from another child's.

✓ **Rehearse.** Practice communicating what your child needs in order to keep him or her safe.

✓ **Be a problem solver. Be proactive.** Explain the needs of your child and clearly list (in writing) what *is* safe as well as what *is not* safe.

✓ **Face-to-face meetings work best.** Prepare for every meeting and bring a supportive friend or relative if you feel the encounter may be emotional.

✓ **Plan ahead.** In the fall, sit down with the school nurse, teachers, and administrators. Thank them for keeping your child safe, and discuss the upcoming year. Have them agree to meet with you again in the spring before the following year.

✓ **Trust your instincts.** As a parent, many times you are put in uncomfortable situations. If you don't feel it's safe at a friend's home for a play date, kindly decline, invite them to your home, or request that you or a chaperone be present. Once you've set the ground rules for a play date, people usually are happy to accommodate.

✓ **Educate your friends (with humor).** Don't assume that other people know about food allergies, and don't be afraid to start from basics. For example, you can say something like "Yes, I am now the peanut police. I have to tell people to wipe their table down, even though it is probably perfectly clean." You can educate people and still keep the tone light and conversational.

✓ **Help your child educate friends.** Friends can be your child's strongest advocates and most valuable safety nets.

✓ **Help educate other caregivers.** Talk to your doctor and find out what precautions are medically necessary to keep your child safe. When talking to other caregivers, use the term, "this is what is medically necessary for my child." This takes the onus off you and puts it where the focus should be, on what the child needs.

✓ **Start from scratch.** Make yourself familiar with as many reputable websites (see Resources) relating to food allergy as possible. Soon enough, you will know what is helpful and what is not.

✓ **Find friends for your child who also have food allergies.** It is good for them (and you) to know they are not alone. Consider having your young food-allergic child meet an older food-allergic child that he or she *may* see as a mentor.

✓ **Provide your child with opportunities to be his or her own advocate.** Have her read a label and tell you whether it is safe. Let him order at a restaurant and explain his allergy.

✓ **Find a support group in your area.** There is strength and knowledge in numbers. People who utilize social support seem to adjust better than those who try to deal with stressful situations in isolation.

✓ **Anyone can be politically active.** Make sure your political representative knows food allergy is important to you.

✓ **When you find a good idea, share it.**

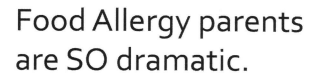
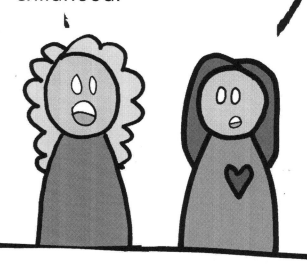

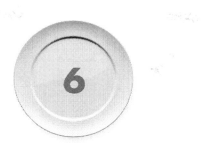

PUBLIC POLICY

food allergy polices ('pɒləsi) *n.* Plans of action adopted and pursued by the government or school or other social group to assist in the management of food allergy and anaphylaxis.

The Food Allergen Labeling and Consumer Protection Act of 2004 requires proper labeling of major allergens on foods. However, it does not require food manufacturers to label all allergens, such as sesame seed. This is concerning, as sesame is among the top 10 most common allergens in children and frequently elicits severe reactions.[1]

Often the public may oppose specific *food allergy policies* in schools.[4,5] Parents of children without food allergy sometimes oppose peanut bans and special lunch tables for food-allergic children.[4,5] This is probably due to a lack of knowledge of the life-threatening nature of food allergy and a focus on the personal implications of accommodations. Parents of children without food allergy may not be aware of the relative ease of working out a win-win solution. Improved public awareness of the challenges faced by food-allergic children may help school-based food allergy policies gain support.

As of 2012, 18 states (Arizona, California, Colorado, Connecticut, Illinois, Maryland, Massachusetts, Mississippi, Missouri, New Jersey, New York, Ohio, Rhode Island, Tennessee, Texas, Vermont, Washington, and West Virginia) have school-based food allergy policies or guidelines. Several public and private schools have banned peanuts, but the practicality and usefulness of such policies is still uncertain. Nationally, President Barack Obama signed the Food Allergy and Anaphylaxis Management Act into law on January 4, 2011; this legislation orders the development of a voluntary policy to manage food allergy and anaphylactic risk in schools.

• • •

"The disparity regarding food allergy management policies between places that care for children, such as schools and camps, is astounding. I have found certain preschools to be very accommodating and responsive while others seem clueless."

• • •

"A mistake could be a lesson learned, but having a protocol on campus and a planned medical plan incorporated in campus response would be a lifesaver."

• • •

"It is amazing what we can do when we work together. I have learned that even the individual has a voice that can help increase awareness at the national level. By uniting and working together, we can change community awareness and policies to help support our children (and patients). Laws protecting our children are sweeping the country, and we must keep the momentum going and focus on a common goal: the health and safety of children with food allergies."

• • •

"I think our schools need to eliminate foods containing peanuts from the menu so parents have comfort in knowing their child will not be at risk when eating lunch at school. I think better education should be provided to our daycares and schools on food allergies and the severity of these allergies."

• • •

"My six-year-old daughter has a severe peanut allergy. She attends an elementary school where they have a 'peanut-free' table that is monitored by adults. We have been 100 percent exposure-free at this wonderful school."

• • •

"I think there should be a mandated policy for public schools that if someone has a severe allergy to a food that that food be banned from the classroom."

• • •

"It is the final two weeks of school at a private school with no way to legally force protections for my children [for example, through a 504 plan]. The food in every class and the refusal to protect and accommodate has made the anxiety level sky-high this past week. Classrooms need to go food-free for the health and safety of all children."

• • •

"I was buying Aunt Jemima pancake mix for my milk-allergic children as always and after the food labeling bill took effect, [the label] suddenly said 'manufactured in a facility that also contains milk and egg.' I had to think twice about using it. I switched to Bisquick."

• • •

"I think different communities respond to food allergies very differently. Different school districts have dramatically different policies. Parents of children with food allergies need to be sensitive to the dynamics of their own community and try to be positive change agents within the constraints they face. I think the food allergy experts can help by providing clear information that explains the increasing prevalence of food allergies and the serious implications of exposure to a food allergen for an individual who is allergic."

• • •

"It is frustrating that products that I have eaten all of my life now have a warning that they 'may' contain peanuts. We went from one extreme to the other. It would be nice if products made without peanuts could have their own equipment so people with food allergies could eat everything that they are not allergic to without worrying."

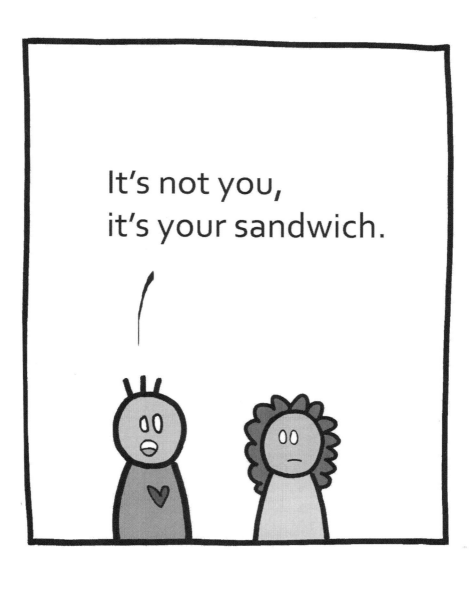

PART TWO: RELATIONSHIPS

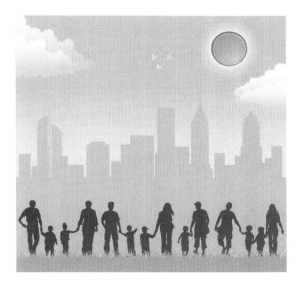

Most parents are *worried* by others' *lack of concern* for their child's food allergy

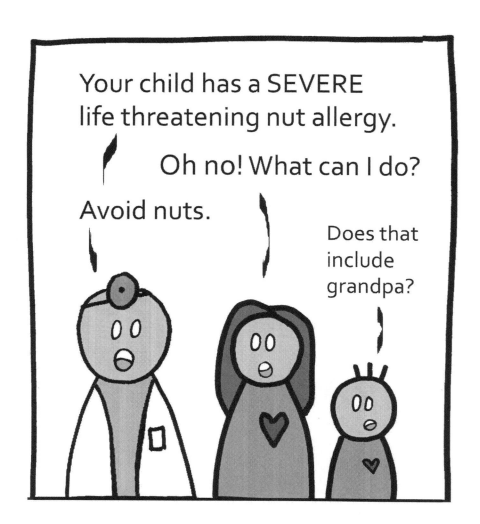

SUPPORT SYSTEMS

There are many misconceptions surrounding food allergy.[3-6] Many people do not believe that food allergy is a serious problem and are not aware that there is no cure for food allergy.[3,4] These misconceptions may lead some people to resent children with food allergy, especially when their own child is directly affected—for example, if their child is no longer allowed to bring peanut butter and jelly to school.

The truth is, without a cure or preventive medicine, a child with food allergy may end up hospitalized, and could even die, if he or she is exposed to an allergenic food. Furthermore, since food is such a big part of everything we do, avoiding allergenic food is not easy for families of children with food allergy. Families affected by food allergies desperately need the support, care, and empathy of people around them. *Support* is vital for a child with food allergy to live to his or her full potential.

• • •

"I have been more troubled this week by my daughter's allergies due to a reaction she had this week that is unexplained. The lack of a local support group has greatly affected how well we cope with her allergies in times of difficulty."

• • •

"Thank God for support groups is all I can say, because the medical establishment isn't something that is helping me right now."

• • •

"My biggest challenge is giving my 11-year-old more experiences being away from Mom. I'd like him to gain more independence from me, but it has to be gradual so I can help him build a safety network."

• • •

"Our egg-allergic son is eight months old. Right now, it is very easy to protect him, and I feel there is a lot of awareness and respect around his condition."

• • •

"In the groups that I have had the honor of being involved in, from both the facilitator and the parent perspective, exchanging common challenges and triumphs is incredibly comforting and empowering. Watching the kids light up when they see others who also need to do things a bit differently than kids without food allergies is inspiring."

At first, you avoid the food. Eventually, you avoid the people who keep MAKING the food you avoid.

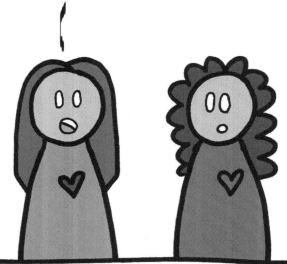

MARRIAGE AND RELATIONSHIPS

One in four parents reported that food allergy caused a strain on their marriage or primary relationship.[5] Marital strain is often seen whenever a child is dealing with a chronic medical condition. Tension and conflict are prominent due to differences in parenting philosophy and practice.[3] Although the following attributes can be experienced by either parent, we found mothers tend to shelter their children from the smallest possible risk, whereas fathers often wish to expand their children's life experiences as much as possible.[3] Mothers are also more likely than fathers to be concerned with a food-allergic child's nutrition, as most of the mothers are in charge of the day-to-day meal preparation.[3] Some mothers even stop working outside the home to keep their children safe.[2] Accordingly, mothers seem to experience a stronger negative impact on their social, emotional, and mental well-being than fathers do.

• • •

"I try to give teaching tools that people can share with the other parent or relative who may not understand certain principles of prevention and preparedness or who was not present at the visit with me. By giving parents these tools, I hope to take the relationship dynamics out of the situation and replace them with facts. Early on, after my son's reaction, my wife and I reviewed basic food allergy management together and quickly got on the same page."

• • •

"Food allergy is the one area in our marriage that arguments come up, because I do not think I am aware of the amount of stress that it creates for her. I think we experience stress in different ways, but I think the fundamental difference is that she feels the day-to-day responsibilities, due to the fact that she is there and she is making those decisions."

• • •

"I worry the most when she is with her father. He doesn't believe that she is allergic."

• • •

"My husband and I work very hard together to make our daughter's milk/dairy allergy a nonissue in her life. We provide alternate food at birthday parties, etc., so she doesn't miss out on anything."

• • •

"I am going through a divorce because my husband doesn't believe our son's allergies are that serious. I will be going to court soon and worry that the court will grant visitation of my son to my husband, who has no regard for his health and well-being. My husband lives with his parents, who also do not believe that my son's allergies are serious. They have not allergy-proofed their house and do not plan to do so. I can only continue to try to educate the courts about the seriousness of food allergies and also pray that someone will care enough to safeguard my son's life."

• • •

"My husband is an optimist and avoids pain, but he is not the primary caregiver and does not always label his feelings as I would. He would say that he is constantly aware."

• • •

"Milk and cheesy things are favorites of my husband's, and he is not going to give them up. He is not going to give them up regardless that they are life-threatening to our child. So milk is in the house, and I follow my husband around and clean up after him. It has caused a huge marital strain."

• • •

"I've spent 50 percent of my time managing my child's food allergies and the other 50 percent managing my husband's disbelief of the situation. The problem is, if you are managing the situation and have no negative effects, the family seems to think it's not a problem, even though our child's test confirms that he has a severe condition."

• • •

"My wife is much more into 100 percent prevention all the time, and I am much more into trying to maximize what my son can do. I am trying to figure out what that limit is so that he can do the most he could possibly do, whereas she is much more in tune to 'Let's not take a chance at all' and 'I do not want to put my son in danger.'"

TIPS

"Don't find fault. Find a remedy."
- Henry Ford

✓ **Both parents and extended family may benefit from being present at the doctor's office during the diagnosis.** When delivered by a doctor, the news seems to carry more weight with all involved.

✓ **Counseling can be very helpful** (religious or professional) in resolving issues related to different opinions about caring for a child with food allergy.

✓ **Don't forget to compliment your spouse** when he or she does something positive with regards to your child's food allergy. Reinforcing what is positive is a great way to start working together as a couple.

✓ **If you and your spouse have different ideas about food allergies, consult with your allergist together.**

✓ **If your child has an allergic reaction, consider taking photographs or a video of your child** (after first ensuring their health and safety). Sometimes a spouse or family member who does not comprehend the seriousness of food-allergic reactions will quickly gain understanding once he or she sees a picture or video of a child experiencing one.

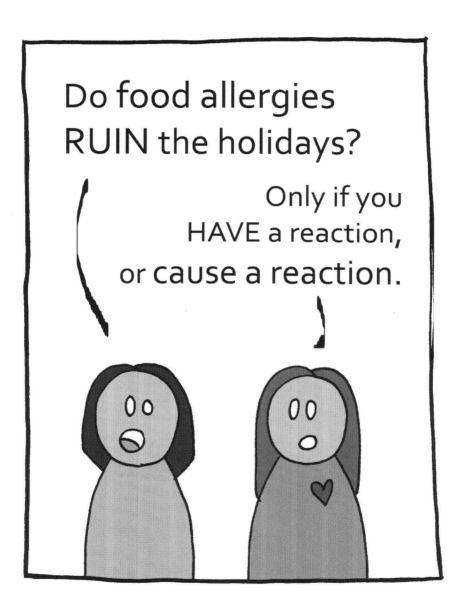

FAMILY

Misunderstanding or disregard for a child's food allergy is a common source of stress among family members.[3] Mothers often feel that extended family dismiss their concerns as "overprotective" or "neurotic" when it comes to a child's food allergy.[3]

Food allergy is very real and life-threatening. A family that understands food allergy, creates a safe, allergen-free environment and learns how to recognize and treat symptoms of a reaction, is a family that supports and advocates for the child. The support, security, confidence, and love for the child are sure to have a strong positive effect on all involved.

• • •

"Most troubling is that my family doesn't seem to understand the seriousness. We've had several family members choose foods with nuts and even serve foods with nuts at family gatherings, making avoidance extremely difficult."

• • •

"Leaving the children at Grandma's is definitely more scary as her advanced age prevents her from understanding the importance of looking at labels, taking it all seriously, recognizing a reaction, and using an EpiPen."

• • •

"My family is very informed and supportive, in part due to my efforts to educate them. More education is needed."

• • •

"I have lots of anxiety due to lack of awareness by other people. I actually had a girlfriend of my father-in-law give my son candy with nuts. Once she realized what she had done, she made him spit it out and then told him to keep it a secret from Mom. He kept the secret for a month. I just found out about it and confronted her. Needless to say, she will never be alone with my children again. I am constantly trying to educate other people about the seriousness of food allergies, and it does not always help."

• • •

"Our home and Grandma's (the only babysitter) home are free of all the allergens that are life-threatening. Our daughter does not visit any other homes."

• • •

"Worrying is constant in our lives. We were diagnosed 10 months ago, and some family members still do not respect the position we are in. Educating some family members has been worse than educating friends."

• • •

"We cannot celebrate normal family holidays like Thanksgiving and Christmas with our family, because they refuse to make it safe for my child. The only way is if I host it every time, which is quite stressful for me. I am fine, but I can tell my daughter feels sad because of it."

• • •

"I would say from my family's standpoint it was very difficult at first for them to understand, and in fact their tendency was to say, 'Well, you are just being neurotic and overprotective, and it is really not an issue.' And frankly, it was almost that they did not want to be inconvenienced by our situation. Therefore it was easy for them to discount it and say that we as the parents were being overprotective."

• • •

"It is easier to produce objective evidence, like printouts from the FAAN website or like this book, than to just tell people about things yourself. Even though I'm a doctor, many of my in-laws just dismiss what I'm saying as being overprotective. So it helps when I have objective evidence to show them."

• • •

"We just spent a week with my extended family, and my oldest sister would pull out peanut butter cookies, peanut butter and jelly sandwiches, and Reese's peanut butter cups nearly every day to feed to her young grandchildren. Whenever this happened, we would excuse ourselves politely and leave. Even her adult children were apologizing for her bad behavior. Honestly, I was a bit surprised by this because several years ago she had apologized to me for not taking my daughter's allergies seriously. Apparently, she still doesn't."

TIPS

"In family life, love is the oil that eases friction, the cement that binds closer together, and the music that brings harmony."
- Eva Burrows

✓ **Provide your family with educational resources about food allergy** such as this book.

✓ **Show your family the educational videos and food allergy awareness modules on the Food Allergy Initiative website and AllergyHome website** (see Resources).

✓ **Take your family to your next visit with your doctor or to a support group meeting.** If your family members cannot come to the doctor's office, ask your doctor if he or she might be willing to provide information for you to give them.

✓ **If possible, plan a time to sit down and tell your family about what actually led to your child's diagnosis.** Ask them not to interrupt you, and discuss the actual symptoms your child experienced. Since it can be difficult to recount these experiences, see if someone you trust will come with you when you talk to your family.

✓ **Trust your parenting style.** If there are family members who do not understand the seriousness of your child's allergies, remember that your child's safety comes first.

✓ Going to educational conferences, or watching webinars as well as going to advocacy walks or support group meetings may help the entire family.

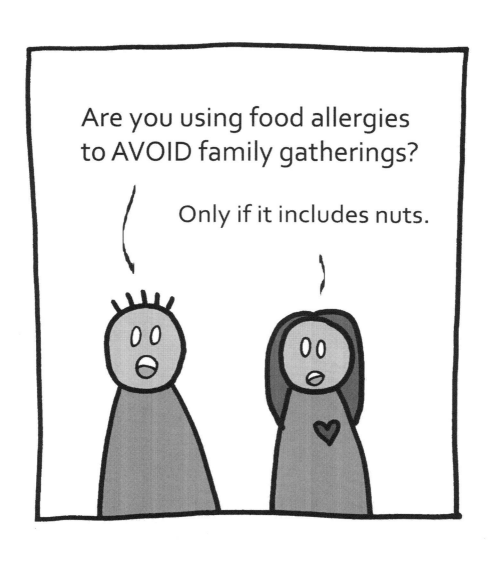

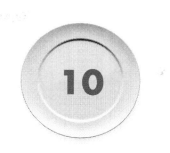

10

FRIENDS

Friends are a critical part of a child's life and development. For a child with food allergy, peer support is even more important to keep the child from feeling different and taking risks.

Almost half of all parents with food-allergic children experience hostility from other parents when trying to accommodate their child's food allergy.[5] An example of hostility includes parents wanting their children to be able to bring peanut butter sandwiches to school.[5] Often this hostility comes from a lack of knowledge of the seriousness and life-threatening nature of food allergy.

Often friends fear not being able to make a celebration safe and therefore do not invite a food-allergic child. This isolates the child and family. Many friends also feel that parents are being overprotective and initiating rules that are not in their own families' best interest, like banning certain foods from the classroom or camp. Addressing these issues may be as simple as educating others about the child's food allergy.

Friends can also be powerful advocates of children with food allergy. For example, a child's friend can show support by asking if a food has a possible allergen to protect the food-allergic friend. Without this type of peer support, a food-allergic child can become isolated and bullied. With this support, a food-allergic child can become confident and live a happier and healthier life.

• • •

"I find the communication with friends and family more stressful than with strangers. I feel like friends and family are quick to put me at ease, so they say they understand yet don't change their behavior and are careless with food preparation."

• • •

"We find that the friends' parents are great about the whole thing when I make them aware of it."

• • •

"We have been dealing with these food allergies since they were 17 months old and have just learned what things they can and can't have. They are also very good at telling their friends or reminding them. The friends are now on board and are probably more concerned about my children getting something they can't have and are watching out for them as well."

• • •

"It is other parents' ignorance or indifference that is the most troubling, because many continue to pack their child's lunch or snack with nut products, despite warnings not to do so. If only other parents would understand that packing items like that makes it dangerous for other children in the group, I would feel a lot better."

• • •

"We are lucky to have a wonderful support system in our neighborhood, so play dates among the three families are worry-free."

• • •

"We try to emphasize self-reliance. We try to teach our son that while we are delighted when our friends make accommodations for us, we are not hurt or disappointed when we need take the lead on providing his own safe food."

• • •

"Our true friends won't set out a bowl of nuts when they have a party that includes our kids. They genuinely care that you feel comfortable and don't have to worry the whole time you're at the party."

• • •

"If we're going into a new situation with people we don't know well, we always make sure they are aware of the allergies beforehand and we carry cotton gloves in her medicine bag. These have been especially useful when we've been around young children who are always putting their fingers in their mouths."

TIPS

"Friends are the family we choose for ourselves."
- Edna Buchanan

✓ **Sharing stories and resources with other food-allergic parents forms a special bond** and often leads to new and supportive friendships.

✓ **Be a role model for other parents.** For example, when sending birthday party invitations, use wording like "Please let me know if any of your kids have special needs I should know about, including food allergies." Parents who have not thought about it might suddenly be prompted to think about kids with special needs.

✓ **Treat your friends as you would your family in terms of education.**

    o   Provide your friends with educational resources about food allergy, such as this book.

    o   Show your friends the educational videos and food allergy awareness modules on the Food Allergy Initiative and Food Allergy & Anaphylaxis Network websites and the AllergyHome websites (see Resources).

    o   Take your friends to your next visit with your doctor or to a support group meeting.

✓ For others that don't have food allergies, I challenge them to try to avoid milk, eggs, tree nuts, and peanuts for an entire week. Only when they walk in our shoes will they even begin to appreciate how difficult it really is.

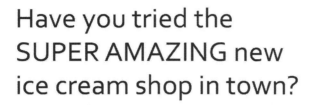

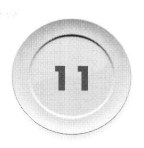

MY DOCTOR

Primary care physicians and allergists play a critical role in the protection of food-allergic children. The primary care physician (pediatrician, family physician, advanced practice nurse, or physician's assistant) is often the first to see a child with food allergy. The allergist (pediatrician or internist who has completed additional training in allergy and immunology) is the physician all children with food allergy should see for further testing, diagnosis, and management. The primary care physician and allergist should work together to develop a plan to care for a child with food allergy.

Many parents, however, are frustrated with difficulties they encounter as they seek out useful guidelines regarding the management of food allergy.[5] Parents may also encounter misinformation, differing opinions, and a lack of food allergy knowledge among physicians.[5]

Primary care physicians themselves express concern about caring for children with food allergy.[6] Recent guidelines on the management of food allergy will assist primary care physicians in improved diagnoses and management of children with food allergy.

• • •

"The allergist in our community did not tell me that there was a support group for people with food allergies, even though he is the medical adviser for the group—this after I was sitting in his office crying after the diagnosis, wondering how in the world I was going to deal with my son's allergies."

• • •

"My allergist feels he will develop a tolerance, but I do worry he won't."

• • •

"My child is almost 14 and was diagnosed when she was one and a half, so we are pretty used to this. She is a level six on the last test she took for peanut. (This year, the doctor made the less-than-heartening comment that he didn't see those scores very often.)"

• • •

"My son was hospitalized at age two with respiratory distress, and even the hospital could not meet his special food needs. We had to bring food from home."

• • •

"I think there was a time when food allergies were a rare thing, and I think pediatricians did not have the same level of concern for it, just like when childhood diabetes was a rare thing. I think there is a bit of a lag and a need for the medical community, especially pediatricians, to step up in terms of their level of understanding of the prevalence of this illness."

• • •

"The last time I was at the doctor's office, a nurse smiled knowingly and said, 'Oh, you used Purell a little too often, huh?' She was alluding to the hygiene hypothesis—the idea that allergies may be related to the use of hand sanitizers and the reduction in exposure of the immune system to normal pathogens, leading it to develop hypersensitivities to nonpathogenic proteins in foods. It reminded me of the old days when we used to think schizophrenia was the outcome of certain maternal behaviors, and mothers were wracked with guilt. I wish people would stop suggesting that if I hadn't washed my hands as much, maybe my kid wouldn't have allergies (especially when it's the same people who told me when my daughter was born premature in November that it was the start of the big respiratory viral season and I needed to be extra cautious to avoid germs)."

TIPS

"He is the best physician who is the most ingenious inspirer of hope."
- Samuel Taylor Coleridge

✓ **Be prepared for your doctor's appointment.** Bring questions in writing, make notes, and review emergency procedures at every appointment. Keep a food log on the kitchen counter. Bring a caregiver to watch your children so you can ask *all* your questions.

✓ **Don't change your child's therapy without telling your physician.**

✓ **Make sure you feel you have good communication with your child's pediatrician and allergist.** If you do not have this, change your doctor.

✓ **Make appointments as suggested by your allergist**, even if you feel nothing has changed.

✓ **Ask your physician and allergist about support groups and other resources.** Remember that food allergy is about emotional adjustment as well as changes in eating.

✓ **Talk to other food allergy families for recommendations** about good physicians.

✓ **If you are questioning the information you have been given, consider getting a second opinion.** There is nothing wrong with getting another opinion regarding your child's health care. You are your child's best, and likely only, health care advocate, and you have every right to explore all your options. This should not hurt your doctor's feelings.

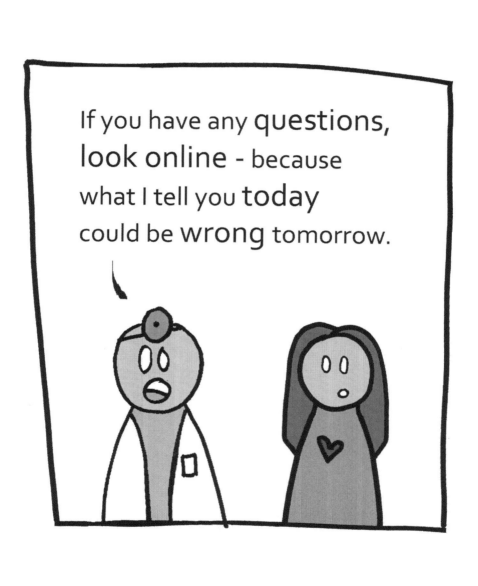

PART THREE: SOCIAL WORLD

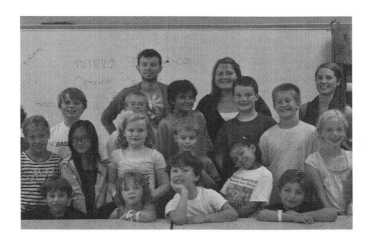

Social interactions place the
biggest burden on caregivers

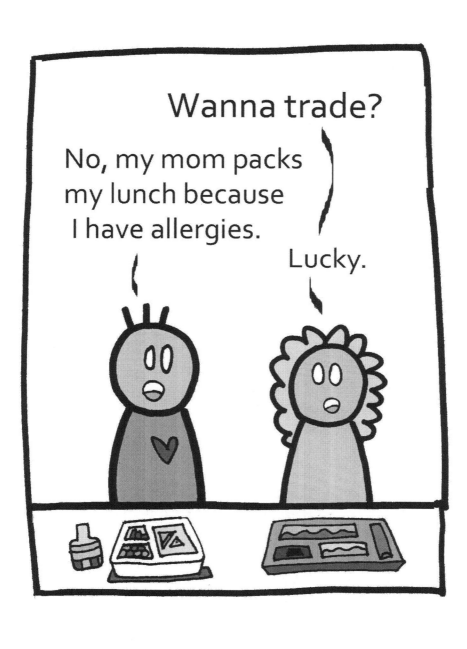

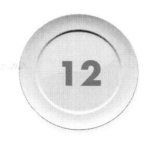

12

DAY CARE AND SCHOOL

Caregivers of children with food allergy express the greatest concern when it comes to school and day care.[2] This concern is very real. Ninety percent of schools report enrolling children with food allergy, with half of these schools reporting a food-induced reaction in the past two years. This is not surprising, given that food is such a common part of a kid's school day, which often includes breakfast, lunch, snacks, and birthday and holiday treats.

Food allergy in children is more common than most people think. One in 13 US children have a food allergy, which means that roughly two kids in every classroom are food-allergic.[1] Peanuts and tree nuts have been found to be two of the most common food allergens.[1] Only one in three peanut- or tree nut-allergic children have medication available at school, and only half of schools with food-allergic students have trained staff who are prepared to treat reactions.[5] Moreover, among children carrying an epinephrine auto-injector at school, only half have a plan for its use in the event of an accidental ingestion.[5]

Schools need uniform food allergy policies to keep affected children safe. Currently, 18 states have school-based food allergy policies or guidelines. Several public and private schools have banned peanuts, but the practicality and usefulness of such policies is still uncertain.

From Parents

"I work from home and homeschool our children because of food allergies. I do not feel schools are adequately trained to handle children with life-threatening allergies."

• • •

"My child had an accidental exposure to peanuts at day care this past week, which increased my concerns again."

• • •

"He is going into school this week—so there is a heightened sense of being 'troubled.' It is primarily while he is under the care of others. We are not concerned when he is with us, just very vigilant."

• • •

"My child has a peanut allergy. Her school, friends, and extended family are all aware of it. My daughter has an EpiPen in her backpack and in the office at school. I am comforted by a high level of awareness around her."

• • •

"My child's school is very uneducated and unwilling to learn about food allergies. I have a horrible feeling in my stomach all day, every day, until I see her when I pick her up after I get out of work."

• • •

"I'm just starting to worry about sending my son to kindergarten in two years. I know it sounds early, but his school doesn't have a peanut-free table and isn't willing to get one at this point. It's the start of a whole new bunch of worries."

• • •

"The school takes my daughter's allergies very seriously, and the nurse is trained in giving an EpiPen, but has never had to do so."

• • •

"I always talk to all the teachers, the school nurse, the principal, and the secretaries to make sure everything is handled correctly with them. We have never had one problem, and the school has been wonderful to help us out with this."

• • •

"In the past week, I began searching for a day care center for my child, who has food allergies. This has been a very difficult experience, recognizing the general lack of awareness and safety for my child's condition."

• • •

"My child cannot attend afterschool activities, because there is no nurse present after school. She is only able to do those activities or go on field trips if I accompany her (again, because the nurse does not go on field trips). Her teacher does not carry an EpiPen——only the nurse or me."

• • •

"He just started preschool this week and *everyone* including the other mommies are tolerant. The teacher encourages phone calls between parents, and my son finally has another little girl with him who has a nut allergy. The school is 100 percent nut-free."

• • •

"Valentine's Day at school didn't go particularly well, which is why it's been troubling this past week. One teacher fed the kids peanut butter candy, with my child right next to another who was eating it. Another teacher passed out candy as a reward that had a peanut warning on it, and my child avoided eating it only because she read the package herself."

• • •

"My kindergarten daughter's class participated in a nice program that provides food for the needy. The whole class went to the cafeteria and assembled peanut butter sandwiches for the morning; it was a wonderful bonding experience and taught important lessons about charity. But my daughter, who is allergic to nuts, was sent to the principal's office to sit by herself during that time. Last night, we got a note saying the kids had enjoyed it so much that they would be doing the program again the next day; my daughter burst into tears and asked if she could stay home from school. I am now looking into whether I can convince the program to allow me to buy huge crates of SunButter to replace the peanut butter, so that my daughter can participate in the future."

• • •

"The room mother in my daughter's classroom told me that some of the mothers were discussing how sad it was that because of my child's allergy, the school policy was to "deprive" all the kids of having home-baked treats at parties. Apparently, when she took the concern to the school administrators, they said it was okay if I baked all the treats myself. I offered to buy treats at a nut-free bakery, since I have a pretty busy job, but she said all the moms really wanted me to home-bake 30 nut-free cupcakes for each of the times we have a class party. I feel like I have to do it, or they'll start to resent my kid."

From Teachers

"As a teacher, I feel like one of the most important aspects of my job is ensuring the safety of every one of my students. For students with allergies, I take a few extra steps to ensure their safety."

• • •

"I have been very fortunate to have parents who are proactive, and immediately seek me out to inform me about their child's medical needs. I appreciate that immensely. It is so important to be able to have an open line of communication with parents. Yes, I receive and read the 504 medical plans or doctor's notes, but nobody knows their child more than the parent, and I value that insight the most."

• • •

"504s and doctor's notices are often very general and vague, and I like to know a more detailed history that fills me in on any prior attacks and what the specific reactions were."

• • •

"I have also noticed how well-informed my students are of their own allergies. They are only five and six, but they know to question whether they can eat unfamiliar foods. It also amazes me how quickly the other students in the class become aware of the allergy and show concern about food safety for their peers."

• • •

"If you have a child with food allergies in your classroom, it is your responsibility to talk to the parents and to the nurse to find out what should happen if there is a problem during the day. When I go on field trips, I take everything the child needs, including their EpiPens, but I have never been shown how to use an EpiPen. I am going to talk to our nurse about having a workshop to educate all of us."

• • •

"Children may be allergic to different foods, and so each year I will usually write all of the parents to tell them we are dealing with a food allergy. Should I have a child that is allergic to eggs, I ask the parents if we can work around this and bring in treats without eggs for the year. I tell them that I think this is a part of working on kind-ness and inclusivity to make our world a better place."

• • •

"Our school is not peanut-free, but the school-made lunches are. This makes lunchtime in the cafeteria tricky, because students who bring in lunches packed at home may bring in food that contains or has touched ingredients that other students are allergic to. I always notice where the students with allergies are sitting and what the students seated near them are eating. Occasionally I will have to ask a student with allergies or a student with food that causes aller-gic reactions to move to another place at the table. I am sensitive to my students' feelings, so if I ask a student to switch seats, I make sure to explain the situation and allow them to move with some friends. Students with allergies should not feel like outcasts, and students that can eat foods that cause other students to have allergic reactions should not feel bad about their lunches. I have found my kindergarten students are always very concerned about the well-being of their peers and learn quickly not to share food and to be aware of allergies."

• • •

"I had to use the EpiPen last year on a student, and I think it saved her life. She was having a reaction that started with hives, so we gave her Benadryl, and then she complained of her throat closing and having trouble breathing. Everyone was panicking, and so I got the EpiPen and gave it to her through her pants. It was easier than I thought it would be, and although so scary, I am so glad I was able to do it."

• • •

"I have been a teacher for over 30 years for elementary school, mainly first or second grade. When I started I had not heard of food allergy, and all kids could bring any food to school and PB and J sandwiches were a favorite. As the years progressed, kids starting coming in allergic to food. Now I carry two bags of meds everywhere I go with the kids and have six children with food allergies in my class. I am so careful to clean carefully and have learned the signs to look out for. I hope we can find a cure soon, as it is really so challenging for the children, their families, and the schools."

TIPS

"I cannot teach anybody anything. I can only make them think."

- Socrates

From one parent to another

✓ **Your child is his or her own best advocate.** From early on, teach your child what he or she can and cannot eat. Test him or her in different situations, such as at restaurants, in cafeterias, and at home. Teach him or her to ask about ingredients. Make it a game to play detective.

✓ **Provide a written emergency action plan to your school.** Make sure that plan is in your child's classroom and is available in case of a substitute teacher.

✓ **Attend field trips and special events in your child's school.** If this is not possible, talk to the teacher about specific risks that each of the field trips may have.

✓ **Consider a child's emotional reaction to food allergy,** not just his or her physical safety. A good metaphor is "relaxed readiness." Encourage your child to enjoy life and participate in school. You (and your child, depending on his or her age) should also be ready and prepared by reading ingredients, asking about the exact ingredients in food, and having an epinephrine auto-injector readily available in all situations.

✓ Ask your child's teacher to include reading and sharing of five books related to food allergy and other chronic conditions, and volunteer to bring them in or come read them with the class.

✓ **Do your best to keep your child included.** Although some situations may not seem fair to you, keep in mind that your child's social well-being is your priority, and try your hardest to make it easy for others to avoid excluding, resenting, or stigmatizing your child.

From one teacher to another

"He who dares to teach must never cease to learn."
- Unknown

✓ **Keep medications accessible in school classrooms.** Place a child's medications, doctor forms, emergency phone numbers, and instructions in a clear Ziploc bag. Write the student's name in large letters, and tape a picture of the student on the outside of the baggie. This works well. In case the teacher is not with the student when he or she has an attack, the adult in charge will be able to identify the student immediately and see all the contents of the bag. All of these bags go in a medical backpack that goes wherever the children go.

✓ **Educate yourself on how to use an epinephrine auto-injector** in case of an emergency. Here is some useful information: (1) you can and should use it through a child's clothes; (2) you never see the needle; (3) aim for the outer thigh; (4) hold it in for *ten* seconds; (5) make sure someone is calling 911; and (6) comfort the child until medical assistance arrives.

✓ **Try to keep some allergy-free treats on hand in the classroom.** Talk to the parents and try to keep something safe that the child enjoys. This helps for those spontaneous food-related events.

✓ **Make sure substitute teachers know about all food-allergic students and what to do in case of a reaction.** On the first page of substitute lesson plans, type, in bold letters that there are students with food allergies in the classroom, and supply the teachers with all information that they need. Also, tape a note to your desk and file cabinets for quick reference. Anyone who walks through the classroom doors needs to be aware.

✓ **Modify lesson plans to ensure certain food materials that may cause allergic reactions are not a part of it.** Always check labels. It is vital for teachers to educate themselves about the steps that must be taken in the event a reaction occurs.

✓ **Always handle the food for the children with food allergies first** when passing out food or treats. Make sure you frequently wash your hands when working with allergenic foods.

✓ **When cleaning desks in a room with children with food allergies, make sure to clean in places where little hands can reach—under and inside the crevices of desks and not just on top.**

✓ **Send a letter to all parents at the beginning of the year letting them know of the food allergies in the classroom and asking them to send only allergen-free treats for birthdays and class parties.** (A sample letter is included in the resources section of this book.)

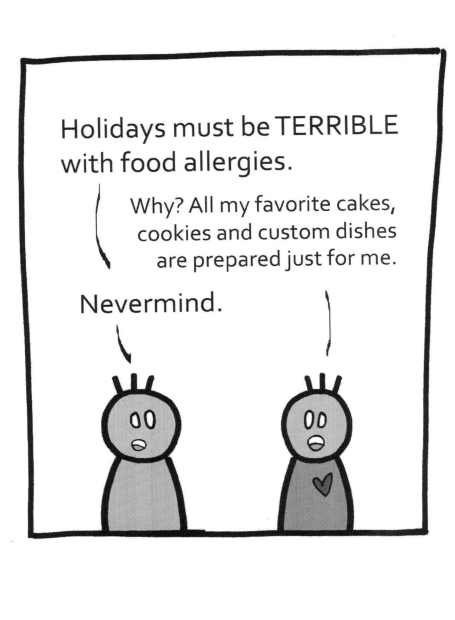

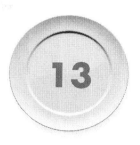

SOCIAL ACTIVITIES

Parents with food-allergic children, whether the allergy is mild or severe, agree that social interactions cause the greatest stress and burden for the family.[2] Food is a key part of social interactions in our society, which means that parents must constantly assess risk to their child. For kids, being able to play with friends is a key part of life—from play dates to sleepovers, overnight camps to birthday parties. Keeping kids safe in all of these places, where food is bound to be, often proves to be challenging and scary.

• • •

"The fact that my daughter has severe, life-threatening food allergies to egg, milk, soy, peanuts, and tree nuts is *never* not on my mind. I always have to bring food to restaurants, people's houses, functions, parties, everywhere, because the allergies are so severe, a drop can kill her."

• • •

"He has been to two birthday parties in the past week. At one, his right eye got red and swollen. He took Benadryl and was fine. The mom called me—I let him stay because I didn't want to make him feel even more 'different,' but I was at home, nervous, car keys in my hand. *It made me so sad.*"

• • •

"My wife and I try our best to check in with our son during or soon after a social event involving food and remind him how proud we are that he takes such good care of himself. We also ask him how it went and how it felt. He has yet to take us up on the touchy feely stuff, but one day he might. We'll be ready."

• • •

"My son wants to go to our church's sleep-away camp this summer, and I don't know whether he and they are up to the challenge of making sure he is fed safely."

• • •

"Kids get treats all over the place—bus, friends, teachers, visiting people. Most people never think about food allergies."

• • •

"I have a lot of anxiety and sadness about not being able to send her to camps and activities over the summer vacation from school because there is always food involved. The adults in charge are willing to be trained to use the EpiPen, but I feel that they don't fully understand the severity of my daughter's life-threatening allergy."

• • •

"A mom assured me that the cupcakes she was getting for her daughter's birthday party were nut-free and should be fine for my daughter to eat. I was surprised, as I knew of no bakeries in our town that felt they could avoid cross-contamination, so I asked where she had found the cupcakes, and it turned out that she didn't even consider cross-contamination (and this was a bakery where the chef had told me that they routinely reuse mixing bowls, etc.). 'Nut-free' just meant 'not actually containing nuts' to her. She is a very nice woman; she just didn't know that what 'nut-free' means to a nut-allergy parent is a bit more specific than what she thought. As parents, we need to make sure we're using the same language as those around us."

• • •

"Social events involving food are so tough and draining on me, as I must keep my baby safe from touching food or others who are eating."

• • •

"We are planning to send him to an overnight camp in May. He went to the same camp last year, and the staff handled his food issues well. Last year, I was much more concerned before we worked out all the details."

• • •

"We just attended a party/Easter egg hunt with neighbors. We were surrounded by kids eating peanut butter sandwiches and peanut candy. My concern for my child's safety was greater than normal this week."

• • •

"It being Easter week, I have found myself frustrated by making candy choices for her and worrying about whether or not I 'believe' food labels and the automated messages you get when trying to track down information from manufacturers."

• • •

"Food is such an important part of the way we build social relationships that food allergy can be really challenging. It is a tricky balance to ensure that your child is safe without turning her into a social outcast. I worry so much about how she will handle situations when she is older and the gang wants to go out for Indian food, and she can't eat a thing."

• • •

"Although we have learned to adapt, social activities still present the biggest challenge for us in dealing with Ryan's food allergies. Food allergies have taken the spontaneity out of our plans; I always want to be prepared to bring something for my son that is comparable to what will be served where we are going. At least I have become a better cook."

TIPS

"I feel very adventurous. There are so many doors to be opened, and I am not afraid to look behind them."
- Elizabeth Taylor

✓ **Teach your kids that food is not the center of everything.** It is important to model for children that the purpose of social gatherings is for friendship, fun, and conversation.

✓ **Let kids know that everyone has issues that make them special.** Some kids have food allergies; others are shy. Some kids are diabetic or have asthma. Some are great at sports while others are not. Kids need to know that everyone is unique and special, and everyone deals with things in their life that are challenging to them. Consider occasionally reading a food allergy children's book with your child to help reinforce that he or she is not alone and that there are other kids with food allergies.

✓ **Make your house the home where kids want to hang out.** Provide age-appropriate supervision, safe food, and plenty of opportunities for kids to have fun.

✓ **Instead of feeling sorry for your child, try to focus on giving back.** For example, have your kids collect food for a local food pantry. Letting them know that some kids do not have enough to eat can make them feel better about their own situation. Getting involved in local charities and non-food-related volunteer efforts can go a long way toward making your child feel included in the social world.

✓ **Keep a selection of easy, quick recipes.** When you travel to someone else's home, bring a few safe recipes as well as hard-to-find ingredients. If you don't have time to cook, see if there are any foods in the frozen section of your health food or grocery store that are safe, and call manufacturers to verify safe manufacturing.

✓ **Consider the consequences.** Think and rethink when you are considering an activity that may be risky (like purchasing a cookie at a bakery that uses nuts).

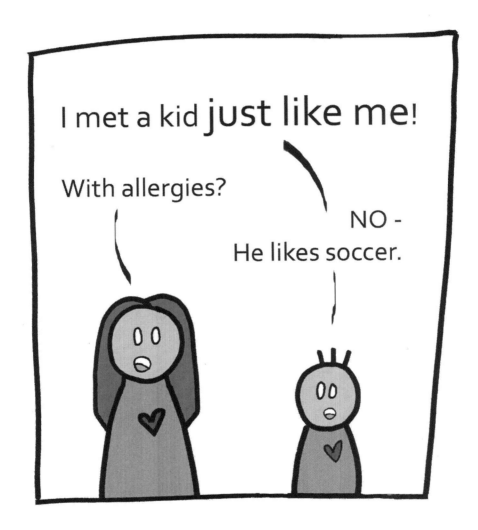

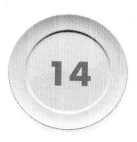

DINING OUT

Dining out is an important social activity for all families. It is a time to relax and enjoy conversations and new foods. For families with food-allergic children, this can be a stressful, anxiety-filled event. It is difficult to know how food is prepared in a restaurant and therefore difficult for children and their families to feel safe. Statistics show that one in four food-allergy-related deaths follow consumption of foods outside the home.

That said, dining out can be fun for everyone if the right precautions are taken. With the Internet, we now have access to websites for many restaurants that post menus and contact information. Look at the menu and select what your child might like so that you have a reference point when you call. Restaurants should be contacted and informed ahead of time, and assurance must be given that the chef can take the proper safety steps. Many restaurants now are aware of the seriousness of food allergy and go out of their way to accommodate food allergy. Support and understanding from all involved will guarantee an enjoyable dining-out experience.

• • •

"I am the chef and owner of a French Bistro and I do not use any nuts as my own children are severely allergic. I still fear them coming to eat in my restaurant, as there is still the potential for cross contamination. Due to my personal experience, I pay close attention to the dietary needs and requests of my customers."

• • •

"We rarely eat out. I've actually been refused service at a restaurant that didn't want to be responsible for cross-contamination."

• • •

"Awareness in eating establishments is increasing throughout the country. Despite increasing awareness and efforts on the part of restaurants, we will continue to need to be vigilant. Always communicate effectively, make safe choices, and always be prepared with emergency medicine."

• • •

"Any time we go anywhere, we have to pack a lunch or quite a lot of snacks so that we don't have to worry about trying to buy something at a restaurant or fast-food place. We try to be prepared every time...but he still had a reaction at the restaurant, and it could be because of the high chair or tables that aren't cleaned properly."

• • •

"There are always cross-contamination concerns. I have tried in restaurants and, too many times, things have happened."

• • •

"We never feed him restaurant food, so his food allergies don't really affect our choice of restaurants. We always pack his food because it's never worth it to risk a reaction."

• • •

"Dining out this week was concerning as my eight-year-old began to have a 'panic attack' after eating a bite of his meal. It was just a reminder to us that this takes an emotional toll on all of us. Fortunately, he was fine. The chef had been diligent about ensuring his meal was safe. However, it just confirmed my feelings that eating at home is the best and safest policy. And we rarely ever do go out anyway."

• • •

"Just last week, I was trying to explain my daughter's food allergy to a waitress, and she seemed very distracted; she was very focused on ensuring that we chose the right wine to go with our meal, and she didn't seem to understand that we really didn't care that much about the wine—we just wanted to make sure the food our daughter got would be safe for her to eat. When she came back with the wine, I asked if she remembered to alert the kitchen regarding the food allergy I had mentioned, and she had no idea what I was talking about. Then she immediately turned her back to me and asked my father how the wine was. She was completely oblivious."

• • •

"I have a life-threatening milk allergy, and this Thanksgiving I opted for the earliest flight into my parents' hometown. I was half-awake and hungry at 5:30 in the morning, and after perusing a fast-food restaurant's menu, I selected a breakfast option I assumed was safe—a bacon and egg bagel sandwich, without the cheese, which is so dangerous for me. The restaurant never mentioned that they buttered the bagel, and only the obvious slathering of the spread stopped me from eating the sandwich."

• • •

"Most food service staff are now getting really good about dealing with allergies. Chain restaurants are the best, in our experience, because they tend to have policies and protocols clearly in place to minimize risks."

TIPS

"There is no sincerer love than the love of food."
- George Bernard Shaw

✓ **Be educated about food preparation.** Talk to your allergist about the risks of cross-contamination.

✓ **Come up with a list of items that are always safe when eating at a restaurant,** but never be complacent – no item is *always* safe. Avoid complex items with sauces; stick with simple, one-ingredient dishes. For example, choose a baked potato, plain rice, or plain noodles. Then bring your own approved sauce, soy butter, or toppings to make the meal more tasty and safe at the same time. But still always ask to make sure the allergic ingredient is not included.

✓ **Speak with the restaurant's manager or chef in person.** Discuss all the foods that must be avoided and then discuss safe options.

✓ **If you find a restaurant that addresses your needs, keep going there and compliment the server, chef, and manager. And spread the word!** Repeat business will breed loyalty on both ends.

✓ **Do not expect that anything is safe anywhere (even if you have eaten there before).** Bring a safe meal that, if necessary, can be easily heated and then properly served for your child so everyone feels included.

✓ **Use listservs and websites as a guide to finding safe restaurants.** However, always call ahead to find out more about the restaurant's ability to meet your child's specific allergy needs.

✓ **Try to eat out during less busy times and on days of the week that restaurants are less crowded.** This decreases the chances of cross-contamination.

✓ **When you are eating out without your child, ask your server what he or she knows about food allergies and cross-contamination.** Use that knowledge to decide if you will take your child to that restaurant in the future.

✓ **Download and carry a chef card** from www.foodallergy.org.

✓ **Call ahead at non-peak hours to discuss safe food options with the Chef.** A phone call ahead can ease a lot of anxiety and uncertainty and result in a smoother ordering and dining experience. It will also let you know if this is not a restaurant you would want to try and therefore eliminate any potentially embarrassing or unsafe situations.

✓ **Go to the manager first and let the manager know that your child has a food allergy.** Many managers will want to take the order themselves and communicate with the kitchen. When you call ahead, check with the chef or manager at the time to see who they would like you to place your order with.

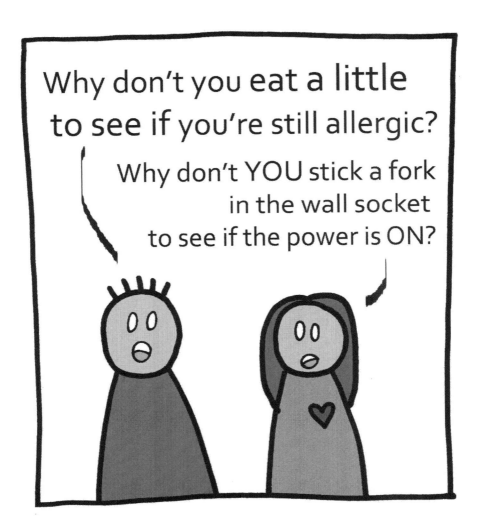

TRAVELING

For families with a food-allergic child, traveling can be a stressful situation. Traveling involves eating out for most meals, often in restaurants unfamiliar to parents, which may be unsafe. It may also mean staying in places contaminated with food residues, which may cause an allergic reaction. However, as with dining out, children with food allergy can enjoy vacation and travel if precautions are taken and everyone involved is supportive and understanding.

• • •

"I have only been on vacation once where we let the chef cook for my daughter. He let me give him a grocery list and watch him cook. He cooked the food in a sectioned-off part of the kitchen, and everyone in the kitchen knew not to touch my daughter's food or cooking utensils."

• • •

"Our daughter flew by herself for the first time this week and is attending a national music conference where meals will be provided. I was extremely worried about her safety. I had to make numerous phone calls to make sure everything from her flight to her eating arrangements would be safe. Even still, I don't know how others will respond to her different needs. I reminded her over and over to ask questions about what she will eat. We worry more about her now that she is venturing out in the world."

• • •

"My son is now fourteen. We travel and eat out a lot, but it is always a huge concern. We try very hard to live a 'normal' life, but there are always incidents that bring us back to the reality that this is a life-long issue. We just returned from Europe, and we had a few occasions that were challenging. I fear every bite he puts in his mouth."

• • •

"Traveling is definitely more complicated now, but with preparation it is doable and so worth it."

• • •

"We are planning a trip overseas (to Italy) for this summer. I am extremely concerned about how to prepare for that and what will happen while we are there regarding food labeling and foods prepared there that he will not be able to eat."

• • •

"We have learned how to spot safe places and those that are likely not safe. When we traveled to Canada last year, we were amazed at how much more the restaurants knew and accommodated compared to restaurants in the US. A couple times, we thought of traveling to Mexico or on a cruise and decided not to because of the food allergy. I'm hopeful that we'll get past that someday. But in the meantime, there are so many places that we haven't been, so we've got plenty to see here in the US."

• • •

"My son is fifteen now and has a life-threatening allergy to milk. He just deals with it. He went to Disneyland on the train yesterday and had trouble finding safe food. He ate fruit and french fries for the day and had a lot of fun. Sure, it would be easier without the allergy, and I would love a cure. But he survives and thrives."

• • •

"We were on vacation this week, and the food issues were very disruptive, as our food options were quite limited where we were."

• • •

"Walt Disney World was great at helping us with his food allergy."

• • •

"On our flight to visit family for Thanksgiving, we had informed the airline of our child's severe nut allergy; this particular carrier's policy is not to serve nuts within three rows of a severely allergic passenger. A man in the row in front of us belligerently excoriated the flight attendant for telling him he could not have nuts. He went on to say, pointedly loudly enough for my five-year-old daughter to hear, that if someone has an allergy like that, they shouldn't be allowed to fly. 'How come some kid's nut allergy has to be my problem?' We clearly have a long way to go in educating others and building a better sense of community."

• • •

"Travel is anything but easy or relaxing for those of us dealing with food allergies on a daily basis. I probably spend a week shopping, cooking, researching and packing for our trips. Do I think it's worth it? Absolutely. I want my daughter to grow up and have the confidence that she's able to navigate the world."

• • •

"Airborne allergies are real, and they can create problems for those who fly with airborne food allergies. Perhaps one day the airlines will learn to be more accommodating. That is my hope."

TIPS

*"All animals except man know that the principle business of life
is to enjoy it."*
- Samuel Butler

✓ **Remember that food is only one aspect of travel.** Get your kids excited about what they are going to see and who they are going to meet. Emphasize that food is only one part of life.

✓ **Have safe treats available for your child.** If possible, make it so that these treats are foods they do not eat on a daily basis, so that there are some food surprises associated with vacation.

✓ **Call the airlines and hotels ahead of time.** Do not be afraid to ask about how they clean rooms or cabins. If you do not get an answer that makes you feel comfortable, try to make other plans. Being aware of policies can also help if another guest or passenger is belligerent about accommodating the needs of an allergic passenger.

✓ **If you can, plan a few days before and after a vacation to relax and take care of yourself.** Cooking and planning can be tiring. Alternatively, if that is not possible, ask a trusted family member or spouse to let you take an hour or two during the vacation to rest and not be solely responsible for food safety. Caregivers need breaks too.

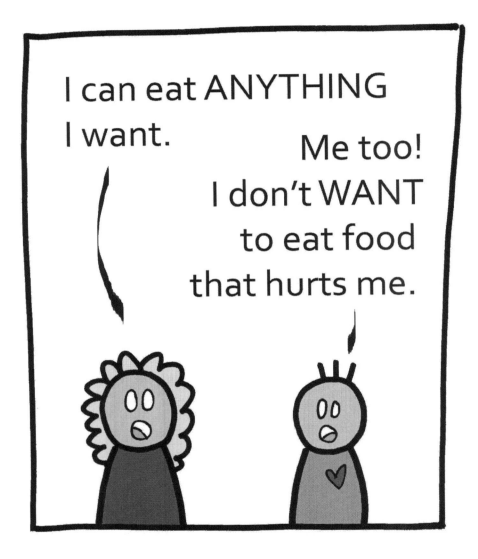

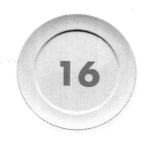

ISOLATION

Food is part of almost everything we do and everywhere we go. Sometimes parents may feel that the only place that their child is truly safe is at home. Parents of children with food allergy, from mild to severe, agree that social interactions cause them the greatest stress.[2] Families may fear leaving the home and may avoid participating in the very social activities that are so important to growing children. With proper precaution and empathy from friends and family, however, parents and children can live a healthy, interactive lifestyle. Helping families feel safe and comfortable in social settings is important for everyone who interacts with food-allergic children.

• • •

"The children's librarian with a local public library refused to structure library programming in such a way that would allow my three-year-old son with food allergy to participate. I had to speak with her supervisor about the library's compliance with the Americans with Disabilities Act of 1990 for them to make accommodations for him."

• • •

"I'm somewhat troubled by the social implications. My six-year-old son rarely gets invited to play dates, and school friends do not join him at the allergy table at lunch."

• • •

"My child is sad and feels different than his peers. He gets anxious around others because he does not know what they have eaten and if he will have a reaction. He doesn't get invited to many birthday parties; we suspect it is because the parents do not want the burden of a child with food allergies at their party."

• • •

"Eating food prepared by others or eating out (and this goes double for potlucks, children's gatherings involving food—in other words, all children's gatherings) is virtually impossible for us. This has a massive impact on our social life."

• • •

The only place I know my food-allergic daughter is truly safe is in our home, *but that isn't living, it's surviving.*"

TIPS

"Be kind, for everyone you meet is fighting a hard battle."
- Plato

✓ **Visualize yourself dealing with a challenging social situation.** Practice what you will say to keep your child safe. Practice delivering an educational message with the appropriate level of seriousness, but also with some humor. Encourage friends and family to ask questions.

✓ **Invite other children to your home to play.** If your child is invited somewhere, go with him or her and try to educate the parents about food allergies. Let your child know how to feel confident and prepared in the event of an emergency. If you feel confident but prepared, he or she will too.

✓ **Start a playgroup for food-allergic children** in your neighborhood or community.

✓ **Volunteer as a family in non-food-related causes and organizations.**

✓ **If you can, volunteer to bring a safe main dish or dessert to parties.** Make sure you explain the importance of avoiding cross-contamination to the host.

✓ **Be a good role model for accommodating kids with special needs.** Food allergy is one issue; other kids have attention, learning, or other health issues. When you are the host, always ask parents if there are special needs you should know about. You might find that other parents follow your good example.

✓ **Eat before or after the party/event or bring your own food to the event.** You may want to go with the child to the event and use this as an opportunity to teach the child what to be aware of. Pitch in and help the parent/host, who can use another set of hands when putting on a party. Your presence usually gives the host a sense of comfort that if an emergency happens, they will not be completely responsible for managing both the party and an emergency. This can also be an informal opportunity to educate about food allergies and show that there is nothing to be afraid of and how allergies can be managed. Lots of people don't invite children with food allergies because they are afraid of the situation and do not know how to handle the allergies.

✓ **Don't let food allergies keep you isolated at home.** Get creative, think outside the box, show your child that they don't have to be a victim to the disease. There are ways to navigate the world safely – start figuring it out together!

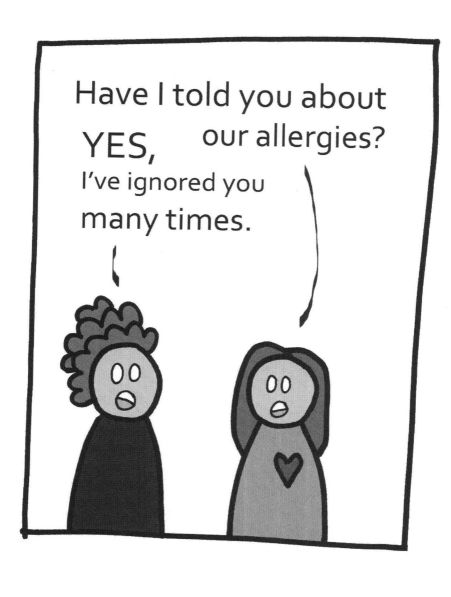

PART FOUR: EVERYDAY

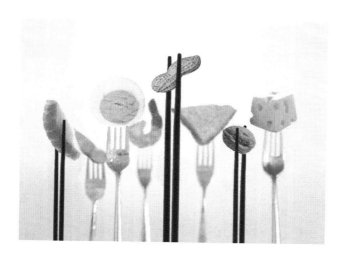

Food allergy can have a *profound* psychological and social impact on the *daily lives* of affected children and their families.

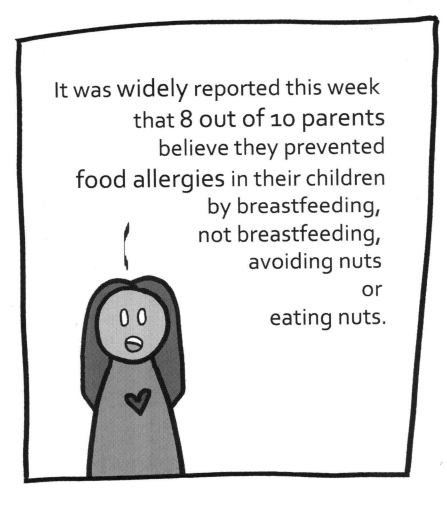

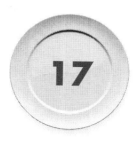

DAILY LIFE

Food allergy is a part of daily life. Daily challenges include attending school, going to restaurants, and visiting friends.[3] Extra time is needed to prepare meals and to take the special precautions needed to leave the home.[2] Developing routines over time helps families adjust.

• • •

"I've tried very hard not to let either the eczema or allergies interfere with normal activities. We never skip an event because of the food; I always bring our own food along."

• • •

"We make significant daily life accommodations for my child's food allergy. We do not mind doing it, but it is a significant investment of time that cannot be used for other activities. The opportunity cost of this lost time is very hard to measure."

• • •

"We do what we have to do to keep our kids safe, like every parent does. We are just more diligent in the food aspect of life. Just seeing a child eating an ice cream cone does give me the creeps, because I know what it can do to my child, even if he touches it. It makes you think of things you would never think of, like if the child is going to wash his hands after eating the ice cream and what he will contaminate if he doesn't."

• • •

"After seven years, I find myself still struggling daily with meal preparation. It's easier than at first, but still a struggle that takes extra time, energy, and thought at every meal."

• • •

"I have set up my three-year-old's life so that I don't have to worry daily. She attends a peanut-free school, and we have extra precautions just in case. I have ruled out what restaurants we don't eat at and where we don't visit (baseball games). She takes her own cupcake to parties, her own Easter eggs at a hunt, and nut-free candy to a Halloween party."

• • •

"Sometimes you can't put a number on the sad or concerned feelings. It's something we deal with every day that is not fully understood by others. It impacts *everything, every day.*"

• • •

"These worries are constant. They don't ever go away and can sometimes become so overwhelming that I feel paralyzed with fear.

It is a daily struggle to provide a 'normal' life for my son while keeping him safe from the food allergens that are so dangerous for him."

• • •

"I am not troubled for several reasons: (1) I cook everything we eat from scratch for general health reasons, so I don't really do anything 'extra' for my one allergic child, and (2) I am at home all the time with my children and am always aware of where they are and what they are eating anyway."

• • •

"My child has had severe food allergies since he was six months old. He's four now, so I don't worry quite as much as I used to. I think you get used to a routine with an allergic child."

• • •

"I think constantly being prepared is how I lessen the anxiety I feel regarding his allergy and including him in different events in our lives."

TIPS

"Life is like a game of cards. The hand that is dealt you represents
determinism; the way you play it is free will."
- Jawaharlal Nehru

✓ **Remember you can only live one moment and one meal at a time.**
   If you focus on your child's entire life, it can feel overwhelming. Focus
   on planning one day, one week at a time.

✓ **Anticipate hidden dangers** by walking in your child's shoes.

✓ **Develop weekly routines for meals.** This could include daily menus
   and safe places to eat outside of home.

✓ **Focus on what is good, right, and going well with your management of food allergies.**

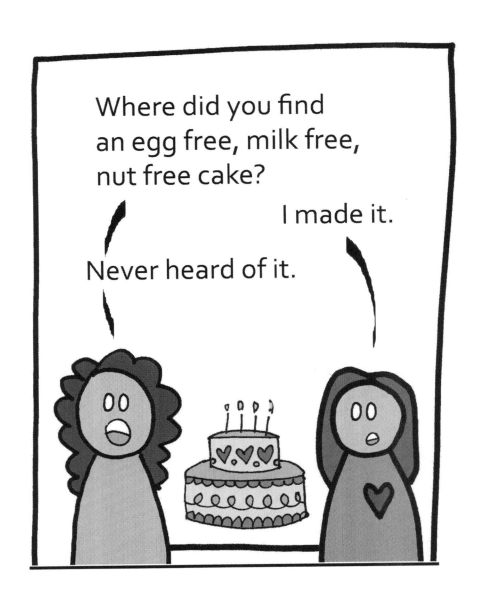

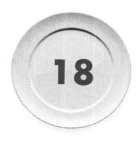

MEALS AND NUTRITION

Allergen avoidance is the first and only line of prevention against food-induced reactions. Children, family, friends, and caregivers must know how to interpret food labels and must be able to identify foods that may contain allergens.

Food labels can be difficult to decipher, even after passage of the recent food-labeling law. Many labels claim that a food "does not contain" certain ingredients, but the food may be processed on equipment that processes the very same allergen. Parents must become familiar with what—exactly—the labeling law mandates and be extra vigilant about what they can and cannot feed their child.

Some caregivers worry about nutritional deficiencies as a result of allergen avoidance; others describe unexpected benefits of living with food allergy, including eating healthier, less-processed foods.[2] Eating healthier, less-processed foods takes time, however, and may mean planning meals in advance and preparing safe meals for outside activities.

• • •

"It was not easy to accommodate the allergies at first, but it has gotten easier as I've learned more and found reliable recipes that she (and the family) likes."

• • •

"My child with food allergies eats extremely healthy (no junk food), so she's okay there."

• • •

"I don't worry about my child's nutrition. It is quite the opposite, in fact. We are more likely to avoid processed and packaged foods now, because of the allergies."

• • •

"I'm not particularly fond of needing to implement avoidance strategies at all times, but it is what it is, and we have no choice. I feel good that we work hard every day at keeping him safe and happy. He's watching everything we do and say and learning from us. Hopefully when he is making his own choices, he'll work just as hard."

• • •

"It's difficult to manage one child with no allergies and one with many severe allergies. I try to balance my three-year-old son's non-allergy diet (although mostly on safe foods too) with keeping my two-year-old daughter safe."

• • •

"The one positive aspect of our daughter's allergies to peanuts, tree nuts, soy, and shellfish is that she in general eats very healthy foods. Since soy is in practically every manufactured food, and we cannot depend on fast-food restaurant staff to be knowledgeable about ingredients and prep practices, she does not eat any fast food or junk food, and very little processed food. I know that she would be eating a ton of this crap if she didn't have any allergies."

• • •

"The past few weeks have become more difficult as my nine-year-old son had braces put on his teeth. Foods that he could eat last month are no longer available because of the braces. This limits our choices, and we are facing new challenges."

• • •

"Premade items are time-consuming to research, and manufacturers aren't always the most gracious or understanding, which makes the task even more upsetting."

• • •

"I prepare snack items and freeze them for birthday parties or school events where food will be served. This helps take away some of the stress on both our family and the family having the function. I have seen an improvement over the last two and a half years on food choices available in traditional grocery stores, and I hope it continues."

• • •

"Many companies are now making products that are nut-free, so grocery shopping is becoming easier all the time."

• • •

"Since I'm the only one who cooks for my daughter, I felt it was important that someone else learn how to do it so I hired a friend who has nut allergies. She comes twice a month to cook for us, and she's learned all of my daughter's favorite dishes. I can't tell you how reassuring it is to know that if something were to happen to me (or if I need a weekend away), my daughter would be taken care of."

TIPS

"Simplicity is the ultimate sophistication."
- Leonardo da Vinci

✓ **Prepare in advance and bring a safe snack for everyone, if appropriate.** Keep a variety of snacks on hand, so you can match what other children may be having.

✓ **Avoid products that *may contain* the food you are trying to avoid.** The US Food Allergy Guidelines suggest avoiding any food with any precautionary or advisory label for your allergen. Always contact the food manufacturer for further information.

✓ **Be prepared for surprises.** Always keep a supply of safe snacks in your freezer and at school. Sometimes you just don't know that there will be a birthday in class or a party after school.

✓ **Read every ingredient label and package *three* times:** when you buy it, when you put it away, and before you serve it. Remember, warnings may not be printed near the ingredients list. Read the label backward if that makes it easier for you to catch every detail. **Teach your child to ask others to read the ingredients until he or she is able to read it.** *If you can't read it, you can't eat it.*

✓ **If a packaged food looks like it may have been repackaged, avoid it.**

131

✓ When talking about a food or meal that may be associated with food allergy, call it by its name. Do not call it a PB and J if it is a soy-butter sandwich.

✓ If there is a particular product that you cannot find at your grocery store, ask to talk to the manager. He or she may be able to order the product for you.

✓ Remember that preparing things from scratch with fewer ingredients may actually be beneficial to your child's health.

✓ Although variety is important, remember that having several key staples in your diet is just fine. Kids do not need to eat different foods every day to survive and thrive.

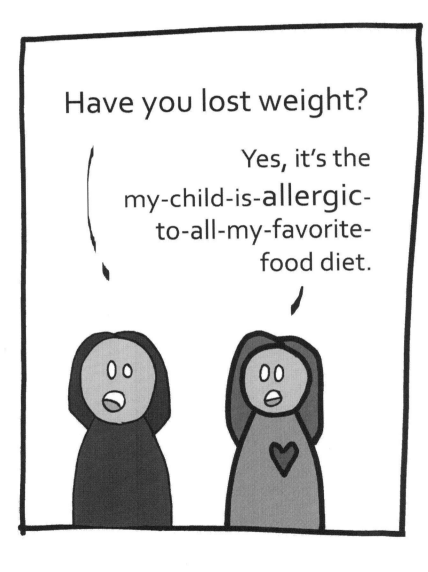

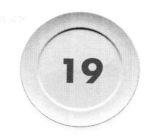

FEELING DIFFERENT

It is understandable that a child with food allergy may at times feel different from his or her peers. While eating for most kids is a carefree activity, a food-allergic child must monitor every food and take special precautions. This may lead to stigmatization, teasing, and even risk-taking behavior. For example, teens with food allergy may take more risks with food to avoid feeling "different."

Many caregivers are concerned about their child's ability to lead a normal life while being safe.[2] Increased awareness and support from peers can make a big difference in the experiences, confidence, and safety of a child with food allergy.

• • •

"Other people just don't 'get it,' as we say. When food is in the classrooms, it creates not only a situation where the food-allergic child is surrounded by potentially harmful substances, but a situation where quite often the food-allergic child is excluded or 'always the one' who is different because of needing an alternative food choice."

• • •

"I have a peanut allergy like my son and have been sad for the things he will miss and the freedom he will lack, such as in traveling to foreign countries. It's an odd thing psychologically to fear food, and it saddens me greatly to think he may ultimately feel that way too."

"My youngest is in pain constantly with his allergies. My children are singled out; they are different. I feel bad for them; I do not wish this hurdle on anyone."

• • •

"I am nervous to think about the future with him not having a normal life. I never want him to feel left out, and I hope to make his allergy not a big deal when he has to have special snacks."

• • •

"Food allergies can make families feel alone and different; it is such a part of our lives that we often don't realize the impact it has."

• • •

"We are sending our child to camp. I am *very* nervous about it, but I can't let his allergy prevent him from being a normal kid."

• • •

"I find that as my children get older (they are now seven and ten), they feel more left out when they can't have the same foods as their friends or when they have to take 'special' foods to birthday parties, etc."

• • •

"This past week my child was to go on a field trip approximately 160 miles away to a dinner theater. We walked into the dinner theater, and two adults at separate times announced in front of a group of his peers that 'oh, you're the one with the peanut allergy.' There is a lack of understanding on the part of some school personnel and on the part of the general public that makes it very difficult to have these kids live a normal life."

TIPS

"Life affords no higher pleasure than that of surmounting difficulties."
- Samuel Johnson

✓ **Focus on your children's strengths.** Provide them with positive reinforcement when they find something they are good at. For example, perhaps your child is a good basketball player, a great reader, enjoys playing the piano, or is wonderful at drawing or games. When your child does well, tell him or her.

✓ **Let your child know that, although food is an important aspect of life, it is not the only aspect of life.** Although food-allergic children are limited in what they can eat, they can still experience the wonders of travel and socializing, just with a little extra planning.

✓ **If possible, invite your child's friends over to your home.** Make your home welcoming and open to friends. This will ease your child's social isolation.

✓ **Let your child know that all people have something that makes them unique.** Although food allergies make your child different, tell him or her that everyone is different in some way, either physically, personality-wise, or in terms of talents and interests.

✓ **Become an extrovert even if you aren't one; it is never too late to grow.** Invite kids to bring allergen-free lunches and sit at the "allergen-free" table. Create a calendar (send it home so moms know when to pack the allergen-free lunch) and turn the table into the "cool" place to sit!

✓ **Overcome the natural tendency to isolate, and instead seek supportive friends and families who are inclusive and who will embrace your uniqueness, gifts, and abilities.** They are there – you just may need to really search and accept a few misfires in the process.

✓ **Talk about your anxiety and recognize that it is normal but also recognize that it needs to be under control for you and for your child.** The world can be perceived as a scary place but you can make it less so with supportive friends, family and professionals, emergency plans, and planning to make everyday things safer.

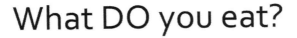

What DO you eat?

Vegetables, fruit, protein,
coconut milk ice cream,
rice milk chocolate...

What about you?

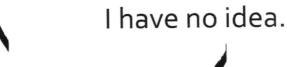

I have no idea.

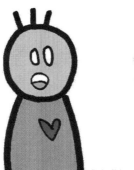
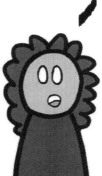

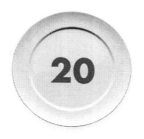

20

THE PARENT'S EMOTIONS

"While we try to teach our children all about life, our children teach us what life is all about."
- Angela Schwindt

Food allergy has been shown to have significant emotional impact on parents. Parents report that the life-threatening nature of food allergy stirs up feelings of fear, guilt, and even paranoia.[3]

Parents who have watched a child experience a life-threatening, food-induced reaction never forget what they witnessed, and they are likely to live in fear of the next event. Parents need care and support from others to know that their child will be safe without their supervision. Plans must be in place in schools, at camps, and in the homes of friends and family.

• • •

"I can only control a small part of our world—our home, and even that takes effort. I struggle between overprotectiveness and vigilance."

• • •

"I just want him to be a typical little boy who doesn't have to worry about getting sick if someone touches him after eating."

• • •

"She is now 12 and has been diagnosed with a severe peanut allergy for over 10 years. Now that she is older, there is less daily anxiety involved, but I am concerned as she gets older and goes out on her own."

• • •

"I worry about accidental exposure and the seriousness of a reaction. My son is only 19 months old, and sometimes I can't sleep at night because I worry."

• • •

"Food allergies are always on your mind. As a parent, it becomes part of your life and routine, but the nagging worry never really goes away. I look at my son, and there are times when I realize just how easily he can be harmed. The hardest part is knowing that something could happen to him when I am not there, and I have to trust that others will respond correctly. I am not sure I could forgive myself if something happened to him when I was not there to protect him. Food allergies take everything that is frightening about being a parent and magnifies it a million times. At the same time, I just can't imagine not having my little boy or the experience of being his mom. *As much as I hate these allergies, I wouldn't change a thing about my little boy.*"

• • •

"I am extremely frightened with my little one's allergy. She was diagnosed two years ago, and it feels like two months ago. I feel like the only people who understand are online, on a blog, in a news story, or have written a survey like this. It's challenging."

• • •

"I live in fear each day, a constant fear that my daughter will lose her life to her food allergies. The fear consumes me. Sometimes it is unbearable."

• • •

"I think it is really important that we remember that these are children who have food allergies rather than let food allergies define our children."

• • •

"I never imagined feeling this much anxiety. Ignorance of others...is the problem. It's not an allergy where you sneeze...it can be fatal!"

• • •

"When he was two, the anxiety and sadness of dealing with his condition became overwhelming for me. ...I was diagnosed with clinical depression and anxiety disorder. I have taken prescription anti-depressant and anti-anxiety medications since then. Sometimes I feel angry or 'burned-out.' I feel disappointed that he can't enjoy something as simple as an ice cream cone or Halloween candy."

• • •

"Every day is a concern, thinking that someone will come in contact with my three-year-old and make him react. It is my worst fear, and I am sure that that fear will never go away."

• • •

"My biggest concern is my son being near others who are eating unsafe things for him. It is the one thing that I cannot control. It makes us very vulnerable."

• • •

"It is a constant level of awareness and vigilance. It is an undercurrent of sadness. It precludes and prevents certain group activities. It is constant anxiety that we try not to give in to and focus on, but instead focus on positive successes. There are fleeting panic attacks and anxiety rushes that I suppress and mental exercises that I perform to combat depression and anger. We laugh, play, hope, scold, do homework, get sick, do sports, etc., like 'normal' families but always with an awareness, whether spoken or unspoken."

• • •

"It is important to remember your whole child, not just their allergies. I try to be as careful as I can, and then just enjoy my child and let the rest go."

• • •

"At times, fear for my son is overwhelming, and I become depressed. Most of the time, I feel we are very prepared for anything and feel he is safe."

• • •

"We learn to live with the constant fear that our child could at any moment be seriously ill or die from his food allergies. At times, I view foods as loaded with *guns*."

• • •

"The possibility of accidental exposures that cause anaphylaxis are almost too much to bear as a mother. It is such a difficult life to live."

• • •

"Every day without an allergic reaction for my son I feel is a gift, and I sigh out of relief. Then the fear starts all over again the next day. Everyone always comments on how hard it must be, but they have no idea that at times you just want to cry because you don't know what to feed your child. Every birthday that goes by, as my son makes a wish and blows out his candles, I wish that someday he will 'outgrow' his food allergies and we can take that last sigh of relief."

• • •

"It is exhausting when you have a child who can die from food aller-gies—not just get sick, but actually have an anaphylactic attack and die."

• • •

"I worry and am frequently saddened by the lack of awareness and lack of compassion I sometimes encounter among mothers of non-allergic children. After I put my child on the bus or drop him off, I often wait on pins and needles, wondering if the next time I will see him is in the hospital...or worse."

• • •

"Food allergies are life altering. Every day, I am faced with the stress of something happening to my son, who experiences anaphylaxis. Every day I wonder if it is the day when I am not there to intervene."

• • •

"It was my fortieth birthday, and my husband got my favorite ice cream cake with almonds but also got my daughter's favorite ice cream in a second cake. She helped me blow out the candles and then disappeared into a corner in the crowd. When I found her, she was sad and tearful that her mother, her protector, would have a cake she could not eat. It broke my heart, and I promised her I would never do this again. As a parent and constant supporter of our children, we cannot be the ones making them feel different or left out, and I mistakenly just did that to my own child."

• • •

"At first thought it can be overwhelming to think that my son could actually die from an allergic reaction to food. Looking at the circumstances of these tragedies really helps to put things in perspective and helps to show that the risk can be greatly minimized by implementing food allergy management. We teach our children to buckle up, look both ways before they cross the street, seek shelter during lightning storms, and other strategies to decrease risk of injury or death. We also teach our children with food allergies the principles of prevention and emergency preparedness."

TIPS

✓ **Trust your instincts and be safe rather than sorry.** If a situation feels like it will be overwhelming (for example, going to a large wedding with a young child with food allergies), it is okay to decline an invitation. It is perfectly fine to be protective of your child—as long as you allow yourself appropriate social outlets.

✓ **Figure out who is supportive of you.** If you have friends who are educated about food or seasonal allergies (or are open to being educated), acknowledge and encourage those friends and nourish their relationships with your child. If people in your life just don't seem to "get it," you may need to refocus your attempts and concentrate on those who are supportive.

✓ **Banish the negative self-talk.** Stop listening to others' criticisms (or your own inner critic) of how you are handling a child with allergies. If you are taking steps to keep your child safe, then you are doing a good job. Concentrate on getting advice from other parents of special-needs children. If other people give you advice, assess their level of expertise on the topic (do they have a child with allergies? are they an expert?), and weigh it accordingly.

✓ **Practice hope.** A useful metaphor is "relaxed readiness," where you are always aware of potential threats (that is what a good parent does in these situations), but you trust your ability to handle them. You have a plan in place for your child's safety, and then you do your best to allow them to enjoy life.

✓ **Let non-allergic siblings know that everyone has something special about them.** Focus on the fact that other children have unique qualities too. It is common for non-allergic children to feel jealous of the attention a sibling might be getting. Focus on ways to include them and make them feel special (for example, they can bake allergy-friendly treats with you). Encourage periodic alone time with a parent based on each child's interests.

✓ **Do not forget to take care of yourself.** You deserve to have at least some time when you do something fun or relaxing. You cannot take care of others if you don't take care of yourself.

✓ **Remember that a child's diagnosis of food allergy can be a traumatic event for the child and the entire family.** The diagnosis may have involved an ambulance or a life-threatening reaction. Specific memories about the diagnosis of the child should be shared with supportive friends and family. If you are unsure if someone will be supportive, remember that you do not need to share all the details of your difficult memories.

✓ **Our children look to us for cues on how to respond to situations.** If we show our anxiety, they will copy our emotions, fears, and anxieties.

✓ **Educate, prepare, and plan for success.** Plan for the best and prepare for the worst. Have an emergency or exit strategy before you go, in case things don't go well.

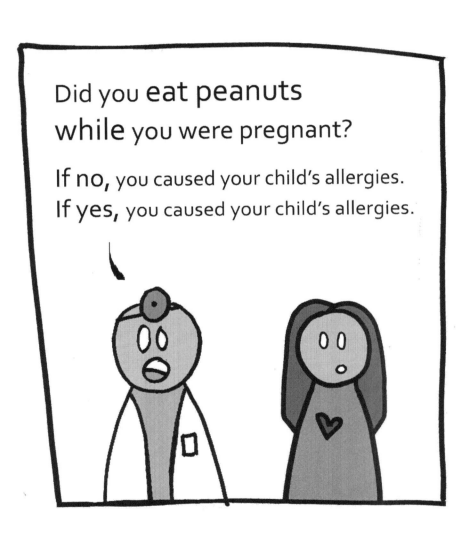

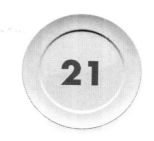

21

THE CHILD'S EMOTIONS

Food allergy affects a child psychologically and socially.[2,3] Children must learn from an early age that they cannot eat freely. They must be taught to ask about ingredients before eating anything offered to them. They learn to bring their own food to events and to avoid one of childhood's greatest pleasures—eating *anything you want.*

A child must be raised with love and confidence—aware of their food allergy but not afraid or embarrassed by it. With support, understanding, and love, a child learns to adjust to his or her food allergy and stay healthy and safe.

• • •

"My son is seven years old and has anaphylaxis to peanut and dairy. This year, he has developed a severe anxiety to eating food at school in particular; he refuses to eat *anything* at school. He will only drink water. He refuses to eat even what I send with him, but he will eat the minute I pick him up in the car. He said he's afraid of having a reaction at school."

• • •

"My five-year-old son is at a point where he is angered and sometimes inconsolable when dealing with parties, lunch, etc. He may need professional help if his anger and questioning—'Why did God make me have these stupid allergies?'—gets any worse. I feel so helpless most of the time."

• • •

"My daughter is seven years old, and she is severely allergic to peanuts, tree nuts, and sesame seeds. She understands what can happen to her, and she has developed anxiety with her allergies. Sometimes she does not even eat in school, because now she eats in the cafeteria with other children. Even though she sits at the peanut-free table, she is worried about other people eating peanut butter sandwiches. It's hard to see your child live with this kind of stress. We have seen a child psychologist for anxiety as well. Especially if there is a new situation, like summer camp, it is very stressful."

• • •

"I know he feels very alone with his condition on campus."

• • •

"My son experiences anxiety when eating foods out of the house and has limited his food choices as a result. He is an extremely picky eater, and I believe that his food allergies have affected the range of foods that he feels comfortable eating and therefore his nutritional intake."

• • •

"At home, I hesitated to give the EpiPen to my son and he said, 'Mommy, be brave.'"

• • •

"I have not found anyone addressing the burden of isolation carried by these children, even with modification. How do we help our children not feel like my eight-year-old, who said, 'My life is horrible'?"

• • •

"My four-year-old son asked for a birthday present on his next birthday. He wants an entire buffet of gluten-free, nut-free, soy-free, and lentil-free foods."

• • •

"We try to remember to praise our son for taking good care of himself. Sometimes it's not easy for him. It is becoming a bit more routine now, but it will probably always take hard work. Every once in a while he surprises us with his acceptance of his difference. Way to go, buddy."

• • •

"My daughter, like many food-allergic children, is wise beyond her years. Her insight and strength amaze us all. How blessed we are to have her in our lives – food allergies and all. I often remind her of this when she gets sad."

TIPS

"The best and most beautiful things in the world cannot be seen or even touched. They must be felt with the heart."
- Helen Keller

✓ **Keep an open line of communication with your children.** Talk about what may or may not happen in their day-to-day lives when you are not with them—even kissing.

✓ **Teach your child to recognize the signs of a serious reaction.**

✓ **Encourage your child to trust his or her instincts if he or she is unsure about a food.**

✓ **Social support is very important, particularly as a child grows older.** Enlist your child's good friends, and teach them the signs of a reaction and how to administer an epinephrine auto-injector. This will help reduce your child's anxiety and will make friends feel more invested in your child's well-being.

✓ **Plan for ways that your child can carry an epinephrine auto-injector at all times,** particularly in social situations. For example, girls can carry purses that they can select to make them feel special. Boys can explore the utility of epinephrine auto-injector carriers. Having clothes with multiple pockets is helpful. Children now always have their phone and keys, so add their epinephrine auto-injector to that list.

✓ As kids start to self-carry their meds, they may actually lose their epinephrine auto-injector if it falls out of their clothes. If you do not get angry with them, the likelihood is increased that they will be sure to keep it with them in the future.

✓ If your child is having high levels of anxiety, seek help from a mental health professional who specializes in cognitive-behavioral therapy or dialectical behavior therapy. As with any chronic medical condition, anxiety and/or depression can occur. These professionals can help your child manage anxiety in small steps, until they feel they can eat safe, predictable foods and feel prepared for rare emergencies.

✓ Consider taking your non-allergic child out to eat the allergenic food outside of your home. It is okay to have ice cream with your non-allergic child. You must help balance the safety and emotional well-being of all your kids.

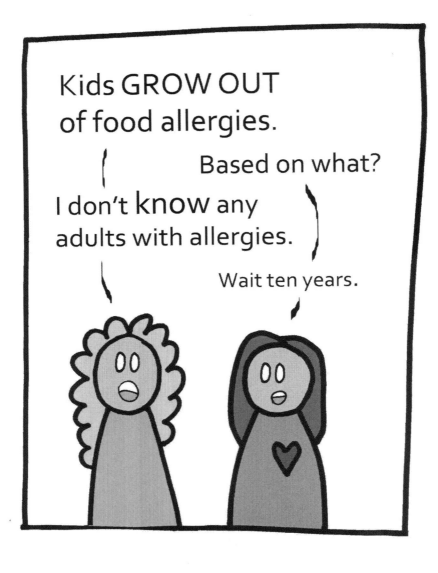

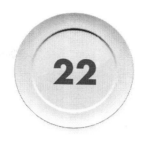

22

TRANSITIONS AND GROWING UP

"Every child is an artist. The problem is how to remain an artist once he grows up."

- Pablo Picasso

As children transition into independent young adults, parents progressively lose control of their actions and food choices. Such transitions occur at multiple points in the child's life and may provoke anxiety.

For most, the first transition is day care or school. A parent must trust other adults in the protection of their child and trust that their child knows the importance of avoidance. As the child grows, the transitions continue, from sleepaway camp to sleepovers and birthdays, from extracurricular activities to first jobs and first dates. For many parents, anxiety peaks with adolescence, when risk-taking behavior and peer pressure reign supreme. A parent must learn to let go and trust their child.

• • •

"My child is 13 and is going into high school next year. My anxiety is growing by the day. He is also about to go on two school trips. Independence is a key issue at this stage, and one that few understand from our perspective. I worry about his ability to mature normally and experience all the beautiful things that lie ahead."

• • •

"With my seven-year-old, my biggest fears are when he takes more control over his life and I am not there, like when he is a teenager."

• • •

"I do worry when my children are elsewhere, especially when they go off to college or travel to foreign countries, in regard to their milk allergies."

• • •

"My message to my kids while young has always been 'We always have your medicine, and you will be safe because a grownup will help you if you tell them you feel funny.'"

• • •

"My son is 16, and we are starting to look into college. He is an amazing student, and I want him to be able to go away to college and live in a dorm. I am fearful, however, about having him eat in a dining hall. Everyone seems to equate milk allergy with lactose intolerance. I know his college years will be challenging for him because of his milk allergy—and anxiety-filled for me."

• • •

"Difficulties arise for me more with my junior high-aged child, who is taking more age-appropriate responsibility (making sure he has his meds) and needs more independence (that's the hard part for Mom)."

• • •

"I have concerns about whether my teen will follow his gluten-free diet at school and friends' houses or 'cheat,' making himself very ill. At school, he will not eat *anything* for fear of getting ill, and then he comes home starving."

• • •

"Now my child is in college and bearing his food allergy alone. The soymilk and plain milk dispensers in the cafeteria were switched in the most recent reaction. The confusion led him to delay his plan, which is immediate epinephrine treatment and calling 911. Instead he sought out the chef, and the chef saved his life."

• • •

"It is always on my mind, but we don't let it rule our lives. It limits eating out, cooking, and parties, but at three, he doesn't know yet what he is missing. I worry more about him as he grows up and feels like he is missing something or gets depressed about his special needs with foods."

• • •

"Since my children are still young, I feel more in control of their destinies. ... As they age, I will worry far more, since they will be more independent."

• • •

"Frankly, I am less concerned about a huge allergic reaction—though it is always in the back of my mind—than I am that this will impact his self-esteem and ability to really experience the world if he does not outgrow the allergy."

• • •

"I feel that we have reached a point where the food allergies are somewhat under control. My children know not to eat food that I haven't approved. I worry more about when they enter the teenage years and engage in riskier behavior and when they go to college."

• • •

"I'm worrying more about peer pressure, since she is a preteen."

• • •

"My son is 16, and we have been living with his allergy since he was little. He reads food labels carefully and doesn't go near anything with peanuts or processed in those machines. It is no longer a 'real' burden for us, because he is careful with what he eats."

TIPS

"If you want to travel fast, you travel alone. If you want to go far, travel with others."
- African proverb

✓ **You are doing a great job when your child has not had a reaction for some time.** Remain vigilant, and use the time to prepare for the next stages of your child's life.

✓ **It is important to let your child know that food allergy is serious but does not define who he or she is or can become.** Be aware, vigilant, and prepared, but still live life. It's a tough balance. You definitely don't want to scare your child—especially a young one.

✓ **If you have a mild to moderate level of anxiety, it is okay to share it with your preteen or teenage child.** However, in addition to your feelings, you should focus on problem solving together and planning for ways to be safe.

✓ **If you have a high level of anxiety that is interfering with your ability to sleep or function during the day, do not discuss it with your child.** You should seek help from a mental health professional to focus on ways to cope with stress and anxiety.

✓ **If your child is older, it might be good to have your physician talk to your child periodically** (in a way that is not overwhelming).

Older kids might need to be reminded of the importance of carrying an epinephrine auto-injector and avoiding food to which they are allergic.

✓ **Plan for today, hope for tomorrow, and don't worry about how they will manage 10 years from now.** Lots can change; focus on today.

✓ **Training for the older child begins at an early age and is a continual process** of slowly turning over responsibilities, as appropriate for their age and maturity level.

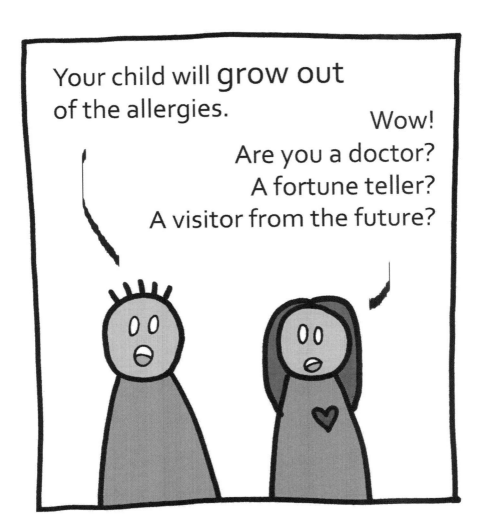

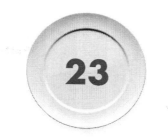

23

SUCCESS STORIES

"Be the change you wish to see in the world."
- Mahatma Gandhi

Although this book describes the challenges of families with food allergy, success is part of everyday life too. With time, support, and education, families learn to adapt to food allergy and not let food allergy define them.

• • •

"We have been living with food allergies for almost 20 years now. We live as normal a lifestyle as possible, taking care to ensure foods are safe to eat. I think it is very important to educate others about food allergies."

• • •

"*Knowledge is power,* and we have learned as much as we can to protect her. Nothing will ever erase the memory of almost losing our child to anaphylactic shock, and we will always have an underlying fear, but we have learned to control obsessing too much over it."

• • •

"When my daughter was diagnosed with her peanut allergy, I was more anxious about allergy concerns than I am now. Keeping informed, scanning the environment, asking the right questions at restaurants and friends' houses, and reading labels comes more naturally now."

• • •

"My child is now nine years old and very responsible with managing her allergies for her young age. This has alleviated some of the stress from when she was a small child."

• • •

"We have been dealing with food allergies for about 10 years. I am comfortable in our routine, and my children are of the age that they will not likely outgrow their current allergies. We have learned to live with and accept them as part of our lives. They know how to take care of themselves quite well now."

• • •

"I have an extremely severe peanut allergy and have had it since I was five. So as his middle-aged mother, I am quite used to living with and dealing with food allergies. Therefore I may not find the problem half as overwhelming as someone who is newly dealing with it."

• • •

"Because my son is 10 years old, I don't have the anxieties I did when he was little. It was a lot more work preparing for trips, visits to friends' houses, and parties. It's gotten easier, but he is more self-sufficient and cautious."

• • •

"The food allergy is always in the back of our minds but does not trouble us greatly, because we are now, after six years, accustomed to the precautions and arrangements that we need to make."

• • •

"Why focus on all these negatives? Food allergies only rule your life if you allow them to. My son leads a perfectly normal life because we don't treat him like he needs to be in a bubble."

• • •

"My son is 13, has multiple life-threatening anaphylactic food allergies on ingestion and skin contact, as well as other medical issues. He is home-tutored along with his younger sister. We are vigilant and well versed in coping with accidental exposure, which is rare. In other words, we have adapted our lives to living as safely and as happily as we can with life-threatening anaphylaxis."

• • •

"We've been living with his allergy for so long that it has become a way of life, and we don't look at it as a burden, just a fact of life. Life is too short to spend it worrying yourself sick. I take the approach that I will train him to look after himself, because ultimately he's the only one that can do it for his lifetime. He cannot rely on others to look after him when he's grown up."

• • •

"We have settled into a routine that involves not bringing food with nuts into our house, sending our son to a school that does not permit nuts, providing alternative treats for birthday parties, etc., so these things do not bother me much now. They did in the beginning though. It has been about two and a half years since he was diagnosed."

• • •

"I think it is easier to be a child with a life-threatening food allergy than a parent of one. I knew I could control what I ate, and I always had empathy for friends who had anaphylactic reactions to bee stings, because they couldn't control when a bee stung them. I realize how hard it must have been for my parents, because they had to empower me to be proactive about my allergies. I was taught at a very young age to speak up for myself, a skill that benefits me today personally and professionally. "

• • •

"It is still a daily challenge to avoid dairy, even after 26 years of living with this allergy. I am constantly questioning menus as well as friends. Even those closest to me forget. But this reality is as much a boon as an inconvenience. I know how to assert myself. I know how to verbalize my wants and needs. My smarter, more confident friends cannot do so as well as I do. It is an invaluable skill, and one I owe to my life-threatening allergy to milk and to my wonderful parents, who taught me well."

• • •

"We are in our ninth year of heightened awareness. This is our new 'normal.'"

FINAL THOUGHTS

"To laugh often, to win the affection of children, to earn the appreciation of honest critics and endure the betrayal of false friends, to appreciate beauty, to find the best in others, to leave the world a bit better, whether by a healthy child, a garden patch...to know even one life has breathed easier because you have lived. This is to have succeeded!"

\- Emerson

I hope this book improves awareness and knowledge of food allergy and highlights the powerful emotions surrounding it. The comics in this book are there to help us laugh, which is so important.

Although food allergy is very real and serious, it is important to remember and thank all the parents, families, teachers, doctors, researchers, friends, and organizations who work so hard to make the world a better place for our kids. This could be anyone from a friend saying she understands, to a teacher proactively helping us avoid allergenic foods in school. It could be a physician teaching us how to use an epinephrine auto-injector or researchers working to find a cure for food allergies.

Hopefully, we can all work together to make this comic a reality. In the next generation, instead of seeing an increase in food allergy, I am confident we will see a decrease along with a cure. This is our wish and goal. Until then, we will continue to cherish our children with food allergy and together help them develop to their full potential.

We would love to hear your thoughts about this book, ideas for future development, personal stories, or whatever you would like to share.

Please write to Dr. Ruchi Gupta at rugupta@luriechildrens.org or to Denise Bunning at info@mochallergies.org.

RESOURCES

There are many personal and commercial sites out there without terms of service, privacy policies, ownership information, and so on. It can be hard for parents to discern reputable websites from questionable ones. Social media has muddied these waters a lot.

Be cautious when you are doing research about food allergies online. Use the following sites or government sponsored websites like MedlinePlus (http://www.nlm.nih.gov/medlineplus/healthyweb-surfing.html) and look to see if any health websites you find ascribe to the Health On the Net (HON) code of conduct.

National and International Organizations

Food Allergy Initiative
515 Madison Ave., Suite 1912
New York, NY 10022
212-207-1974
www.faiusa.org

Food Allergy & Anaphylaxis Network
11781 Lee Jackson Hwy., Suite 160
Fairfax, VA 22033
800-929-4040
www.foodallergy.org

American Academy of Allergy, Asthma and Immunology
555 East Wells Street, Suite 1100
Milwaukee, WI 53202
800-822-2762
www.aaaai.org

American College of Allergy, Asthma and Immunology
85 West Algonquin Road, Suite 550
Arlington Heights, IL 60005
800-842-7777
www.acaai.org

Asthma and Allergy Foundation of America
1233 20th Street, NW, Suite 402
Washington, DC 20036
800-7-ASTHMA
www.aafa.org

Allergy and Asthma Network/Mothers of Asthmatics
3554 Chain Bridge Road, Suite 200
Fairfax, VA 22030-2709
800-878-4403
www.aanma.org

American Academy of Pediatrics
141 Northwest Point Boulevard
Elk Grove Village, IL 60007-1098
847-434-4000
www.aap.org

Academy of Nutrition and Dietetics
120 S. Riverside Plaza, Suite 2000
Chicago, IL 60606
800-877-1600
www.eatright.org

The Elliot and Roslyn Jaffe Food Allergy Institute
Mount Sinai School of Medicine
One Gustave L. Levy Place, Box 1198
New York, NY 10029
212-241-5548
www.mssm.edu/research/programs/jaffe-food-allergy-institute

National Institutes of Health
National Institute of Allergy and Infectious Diseases
6610 Rockledge Drive, MSC 6612
Bethesda, MD 20892
www.niaid.nih.gov

MedicAlert Foundation International
2323 Colorado Ave.
Turlock, CA 95382
888-633-4298
www.medicalert.org

Anaphylaxis Canada
2005 Sheppard Ave. East, Suite 800
Toronto, ONT M2J 5B4, Canada
866-785-5660
www.anaphylaxis.ca

Support and Advocacy Groups

Allergy Moms
www.allergymoms.com

Kids With Food Allergies Foundation
www.kidswithfoodallergies.org

MOCHA
Mothers of Children Having Allergies
www.mochallergies.org

The Allergist Mom
www.theallergistmom.com

The Food Allergy Mama
www.foodallergymama.com

504 Plan Resources

U.S. Department of Education Office for Civil Rights
FAQ for Section 504 Plans
www2.ed.gov/about/offices/list/ocr/504faq.html

Food Allergy Initiative
Search 504 at www.faiusa.org

Food Allergy & Anaphylaxis Network
Search 504 at www.foodallergy.org

Publications

Allergic Living
P.O. Box 1042
Niagara Falls, NY 14304
888-771-7747
www.allergicliving.com

Living Without
800 Connecticut Ave.
Norwalk, CT 06854
800-424-7887
www.livingwithout.com

You will find many allergen-free food and snack companies listed
and advertised in the above-named publications.

Books

Children's Books

Allie the Allergic Elephant by Nicole S. Smith
Taking Food Allergies to School by Ellen Weiner
The BugaBees—Friends with Food Allergies by Amy Recob

Parenting Books

Food Allergies for Dummies by Robert A. Wood, MD
How to Manage Your Child's Life-Threatening Food Allergies by
Linda Marienhoff Coss
The Parent's Guide to Food Allergies by Marianne S. Barber

Cookbooks

Bakin' Without Eggs by Rosemarie Emro
The Divvies Bakery Cookbook by Lori Sandler
The Food Allergy Mama's Baking Book by Kelly Rudnicki
Whole Foods Allergy Cookbook by Cybele Pascal

Other Books

Beyond a Peanut by Dina Clifford
Don't Kill the Birthday Girl: Tales from an Allergic Life by Sandra Beasley
Feeding Eden: The Trials and Triumphs of a Food Allergy Family by Susan Weissman

Check out these websites for additional book recommendations

Food Allergy Bookstore (www.foodallergybooks.com)
FAI's Bookshelf (www.faiusa.org)
FAAN's Books and Booklets (www.foodallergy.org)
Kids with Food Allergies Book Shop (www.kidswithfoodallergies.org)

To view even more fun allergy cartoons, visit
www.FoodAllergyFun.Blogspot.com

Food Allergy Friendly Summer Camps

Anaphylaxis and Food Allergy Association of Minnesota
651-644-5937
www.minnesotafoodallergy.org

Camp Emerson
800-782-3395
www.campemerson.com

Everything Summer
866-995-1122
www.everythingsummer.com

Travel

Walt Disney World, Orlando, Florida
disneyworld.disney.go.com
Special Dietary Requests
disneyworld.disney.go.com/guest-services/special-dietary-requests
Disney's Dining Reservation Center: 407-939-3463

Club Med
www.clubmed.us.com

Reference Chart Comparing Airlines
www.allergicliving.com

AllergySafeTravel
An online travel resource for those with food allergies that identifies hotels with kitchens, health food stores, medical facilities, and restaurants. They also have the latest information on airline travel.
www.allergysafetravel.com

Related Diseases: Celiac, Eosinophilic Esophagitis

American Partnership for Eosinophilic Disorders

P.O. Box 29545
Atlanta, GA 30359
713-493-7749
www.apfed.org

Celiac Sprue Association
P.O. Box 31700
Omaha, NE 68131-0700
877-272-4272
www.csaceliacs.org

CURED Foundation
P.O. Box 32
Lincolnshire, IL 60069
www.curedfoundation.org

University of Chicago Celiac Disease Center
5841 S. Maryland Avenue, Mail Code 4069
Chicago, IL 60637
773-702-7593
www.celiacdisease.net

SAMPLE LETTER FROM A SCHOOL PRINCIPAL

Dear Parents:

You've all read the headlines and seen the news stories: food allergies are a growing concern in schools across America. Millions of children—children who are perfectly healthy and normal in every other way—must watch every single bite they eat or risk suffering a severe or even life-threatening reaction. In fact, food allergies claim an estimated 150 lives and are responsible for more than 125,000 emergency room visits each year. A major health issue such as this must be taken very seriously, and it has always been the policy of this school to make the safety and well-being of our students our top priority.

A student in your child's class has a serious _____ allergy. A child with a serious _____ allergy can suffer a reaction merely by touching a food containing the ingredient. Therefore, we are putting the following safety guidelines into effect:

- Please do not send any foods containing _____ to be eaten as snacks in the classroom. It is fine to send these products for lunch, which is eaten in the cafeteria.

- We will not be doing any classroom projects that involve _____, like bird feeders that contain _____ or art projects using _____ shells. Please do not send any of these projects into the classroom with your child.

- Birthday parties are a special time for children, but can be a difficult time for the food-allergic child. If you would like to send in baked goods, please be careful about the ingredients. Please list the ingredients on the outside of the package, and when

179

preparing "treats" please pay close attention to cross-contamination in your kitchen. To prevent cross-contamination, it is necessary that cooking utensils and preparation surfaces be carefully washed after each food is touched. It would be especially helpful if you could let your child's teacher know a few days ahead of when you'd like to celebrate your child's birthday, so that the food-allergic child can provide his or her own safe treat.

- We will try to keep the food at holiday parties to a minimum. As with birthday parties, we must be extremely careful about the ingredients in all of the food items. Please do not enclose candy or other treats with holiday cards.

- We will keep a box of wipes in the classroom and may request that all children who ate _____ products for lunch use a wipe to clean their hands when they return from the cafeteria. Similarly, if your child ate _____ for breakfast, we would greatly appreciate your making sure that his or her hands are washed with soap and water before leaving for school. Water alone does not do the trick!

This is a learning process for all of us, but we trust that you understand how important it is to respect and adhere to these guidelines. If throughout the course of the year you have any questions or concerns about food-allergy-related issues, please do not hesitate to contact either one of us.

Wishing you and your family a safe and healthy school year.

Sincerely,

[School Principal]   [Classroom Teacher]

Food Allergy Action Plan
Emergency Care Plan

Place Student's Picture Here

Name: _____ D.O.B.: ____ / ____ / ____

Allergy to: _____

Weight: _____ lbs.   **Asthma:** ☐ Yes (higher risk for a severe reaction) ☐ No

Extremely reactive to the following foods: _____
THEREFORE:
☐ If checked, give epinephrine immediately for ANY symptoms if the allergen was *likely* eaten.
☐ If checked, give epinephrine immediately if the allergen was *definitely* eaten, even if no symptoms are noted.

Any SEVERE SYMPTOMS after suspected or known ingestion:

One or more of the following:
LUNG:	Short of breath, wheeze, repetitive cough
HEART:	Pale, blue, faint, weak pulse, dizzy, confused
THROAT:	Tight, hoarse, trouble breathing/swallowing
MOUTH:	Obstructive swelling (tongue and/or lips)
SKIN:	Many hives over body

Or **combination** of symptoms from different body areas:
SKIN:	Hives, itchy rashes, swelling (e.g., eyes, lips)
GUT:	Vomiting, diarrhea, crampy pain

➡
1. **INJECT EPINEPHRINE IMMEDIATELY**
2. Call 911
3. Begin monitoring (see box below)
4. Give additional medications:*
   -Antihistamine
   -Inhaler (bronchodilator) if asthma

*Antihistamines & inhalers/bronchodilators are not to be depended upon to treat a severe reaction (anaphylaxis). USE EPINEPHRINE.

MILD SYMPTOMS ONLY:

MOUTH:	Itchy mouth
SKIN:	A few hives around mouth/face, mild itch
GUT:	Mild nausea/discomfort

➡
1. **GIVE ANTIHISTAMINE**
2. Stay with student; alert healthcare professionals and parent
3. If symptoms progress (see above), USE EPINEPHRINE
4. Begin monitoring (see box below)

Medications/Doses
Epinephrine (brand and dose): _____
Antihistamine (brand and dose): _____
Other (e.g., inhaler-bronchodilator if asthmatic): _____

Monitoring
Stay with student; alert healthcare professionals and parent. Tell rescue squad epinephrine was given; request an ambulance with epinephrine. Note time when epinephrine was administered. A second dose of epinephrine can be given 5 minutes or more after the first if symptoms persist or recur. For a severe reaction, consider keeping student lying on back with legs raised. Treat student even if parents cannot be reached. See back/attached for auto-injection technique.

Parent/Guardian Signature _____ Date _____   Physician/Healthcare Provider Signature _____ Date _____

TURN FORM OVER   Form provided courtesy of the Food Allergy & Anaphylaxis Network (www.foodallergy.org) 9/2011

HAVE YOU...

✓ Talked with your family and explained the situation?

✓ Placed emergency phone numbers (doctors, 911, local children's hospital, etc.) in a central location?

✓ Joined various allergy groups listed in the index to stay in the loop regarding ideas, opinions, and educational resources that other parents have found useful?

✓ Learned to use the epinephrine auto-injector through your physician or a class?

✓ Stocked antihistamines or other necessary medications?

✓ Placed epinephrine auto-injectors and antihistamines in easily reachable locations (school, home—but not in car, as temperatures are unstable)?

✓ Consulted your school to determine their procedures?

✓ Gone through your pantry and cabinets for any potential dangers and removed them from harm's way (if absolute avoidance is necessary)?

✓ Created a food calendar and found nonallergenic replacements?

✓ Researched the allergen-free offerings at your local grocery stores or a health-food alternative?

✓ Shared thoughts, concerns, and fears with a trusted friend (whether allergy related or not)?

REFERENCES

1. Ruchi S. Gupta et al., "The prevalence, severity, and distribution of childhood food allergy in the United States," *Pediatrics* 128, no. 1 (2011): e9-e17.

2. Elizabeth E. Springston et al., "Variations in quality of life among caregivers of food-allergic children," *Annals of Allergy, Asthma & Immunology* 105, no. 4 (2010): 287-294.

3. Ruchi S. Gupta et al., "Food allergy knowledge, attitudes and beliefs: focus groups of parents, physicians and the general public," *BMC Pediatrics* 8, no. 36 (2008).

4. Ruchi S. Gupta et al., "Food allergy knowledge, attitudes, and beliefs in the United States," *Annals of Allergy, Asthma & Immunology* 103 (2009): 43-50.

5. Ruchi S. Gupta et al., "Food allergy knowledge, attitudes, and beliefs of parents with food-allergic children in the United States," *Pediatric Allergy and Immunology* 21 (2010: 927-34.

6. Ruchi S. Gupta et al., "Food allergy knowledge, attitudes, and beliefs of primary care physicians," *Pediatrics 125* (2010: 126-32.

7. Ruchi S. Gupta et al., "The high economic burden of childhood food allergy in the United States", manuscript in progress.

How To Use
An Epinephrine Auto-Injector

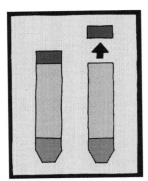 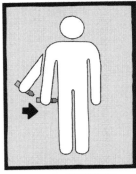 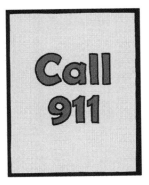

1. Pull off safety cap   2. HOLD FIRMLY on
thigh for 10 seconds

27391212R00110

Made in the USA
Lexington, KY
09 November 2013